Stuffy Nose No More

Who hasn't suffered from a bout of hay fever, felt the sinus congestion of a winter cold or wheezed through an asthma attack? Respiratory distress can range from annoying to life threatening and a good part of modern medicine is devoted to treating its symptoms.

This handy herb guide is chock full of health-enhancing ways to banish malaise of the ears, nose and throat at the first sniffle. Within these pages you will find dietery, herbal and lifestyle remedies for:

- Allergies and Hay Fever
- Asthma
- Bronchitis
- Colds and Flu
- Coughs
- Croup
- Earaches
- Emphysema
- Laryngitis
- Sinus Congestion
- Sore Throat

About the Author

CJ Puotinen has studied with some of America's leading herbalists and is a member of the Herb Research Foundation, the American Herb Association and the Northeast Herbal Association. In addition to magazine and journal articles on health and medicinal herbs, she is the author of *Herbal Teas, Nature's Antiseptics: Tea Tree Oil and Grapefruit Seed Extract*, and *Herbs to Improve Digestion*, all published by Keats Publishing, Inc.

A KEATS GOOD HERB GUIDE

HERBS TO HELP YOU BREATHE FREELY

Herbal remedies for asthma, allergies, sinusitis and other respiratory problems

CJ Puotinen

Keats Publishing, Inc. New Canaan, Connecticut

Herbs to Help You Breathe Freely is intended solely for informational and educational purposes, and not as medical advice. Please consult a medical or health professional if you have questions about your health.

HERBS TO HELP YOU BREATHE FREELY

Copyright © 1996 by CJ Puotinen

All Rights Reserved

No part of this book may be reproduced in any form without the written consent of the publisher.

Library of Congress Cataloging-in-Publication Data

  Puotinen, CJ
    Herbs to help you breathe freely / CJ Puotinen.
      p.   cm.
    Includes bibliographical references and index.
    ISBN 0-87983-741-1
    1. Respiratory organs—Diseases—Diet therapy. 2. Herbs—
  Therapeutic use.
  I. Title.
  RC735.H47P86 1996
  616.2'00461—dc20   96-24278
                                            CIP

Printed in the United States of America

Published by Keats Publishing, Inc.
27 Pine Street (Box 876)
New Canaan, Connecticut 06840-0876

98 97 96   6 5 4 3 2 1

Contents

INTRODUCTION

Who hasn't suffered from a bout of hay fever, felt the sinus congestion of a winter cold or wheezed through an asthma attack? Respiratory distress can be anything from annoying to life threatening, and a good part of modern medicine is devoted to treating its symptoms.

Masking or suppressing a symptom with drugs may bring temporary improvement, but this approach seldom cures a condition. Over time, most pharmaceutical drugs lose their effectiveness or cause adverse side effects while the condition that caused the symptom remains in place. Most American physicians consider the illnesses that cause respiratory distress, such as asthma, allergies and emphysema, to be chronic and incurable. They believe these diseases can't be cured, prevented or reversed, only "managed" by suppressing the symptoms for as long as possible.

Well, that's one point of view. Another is that respiratory illnesses can be prevented, reversed and cured—and that the best therapies treat the cause of an illness as well as its symptoms.

The Holistic Approach

A physician who takes a holistic or "whole body" approach to healing appreciates that a human being is more than a machine. We are conditioned in the industrial West to think of ourselves as cars or robots. Our oil needs changing, our sparkplugs need replacing, our clogged parts need reaming out, our batteries need recharging—and we want it all done immediately with the most refined and purest chemicals available. We have our major medical procedures done in haste and we often repent at leisure. Statistics revealing misdiagnoses, incorrect treatment, detrimental drug reactions, unnecessary procedures, surgical errors, hospital-induced infections and a stunning variety of adverse side effects show that every medical intervention carries hidden costs.

Over the last few decades, a growing number of medical patients, physicians, nurses and researchers have abandoned the mechanical model of allopathic (symptom-treating) medicine and instead look at the whole person. You are more than a diseased lung or string of hay fever sneezes. You are a special individual whose whole exceeds the sum of its parts. Holistic medicine looks at disease not as the simple malfunctioning of mechanical parts to be treated with standard, unvarying protocols; instead, holistic medicine examines the person first and notes the connections between mind, body, spirit, environment, lifestyle, diet, psychological state and symptoms.

Most Americans who suffer from asthma, allergies, emphysema, bronchitis and other respiratory problems are familiar with the orthodox treatments for these maladies. Some for whom the orthodox treatment has been ineffective, or who prefer to avoid its adverse side effects, have turned to alternative therapies for all or part of their treatment. Alternative therapies are growing in popularity for several reasons. They often work as well as or better than their orthodox counterparts; they have few or no adverse side effects; they are often inexpensive and easy to administer at home; they are supported by decades, sometimes centuries, of use and, more recently, rigorous scientific research; and they help place control over one's body and destiny where it rightly belongs, at home with the individual and his or her family.

This review of alternative therapies for respiratory illnesses discusses treatments that are popular around the world, some more widely known than others, all of which have worked to one degree or another for people of all ages, races and backgrounds. There is no single cure for asthma, hay fever, emphysema, bronchitis, the common cold, sinusitis or any other pulmonary illness. Instead, there are many treatments that approach the problem from different perspectives. No treatment works for everyone, but more than one of the following treatments will work for most.

Please note: If you are now taking pharmaceutical drugs for relief from the symptoms of a respiratory disease or infection or if you suffer from a serious illness, it is important to work with a skilled holistic medical practitioner before experimenting with alternative therapies.

An Ounce of Prevention

What are the leading causes of respiratory problems in the U.S. today? Unless you live on a pristine mountaintop in a dry, dust-free house where no one smokes and the wind doesn't blow pollen, they are everywhere: air pollution, cigarettes, second-hand smoke, animal dander, ragweed pollen, tree pollen, grass pollen, yeasts, fungi, cockroaches, chemicals, water pollution, pesticide residues, food preservatives, artificial flavorings and colors, even perfumes and colognes. Don't assume that a pet-free home is free from animal dander. Feather pillows, down comforters and some silk-filled comforters contain dander that commercial cleaning does not remove. Genuine oriental rugs and antique furniture stuffed with animal hair are sources of goat, sheep or camel dander. Wool from undeveloped countries is a common source of sheep dander, unlike domestic wool that is processed to be dander-free. Angora sweaters and inexpensive rabbit "fun furs" are a source of dander that can't be washed away because of the fibers' fragility. Pet birds are a serious source of allergens, not because their feathers are allergenic but because they, too, harbor dander. Even lawns and gardens can be a seasonal source of cattle dander, for it appears in large amounts in cow manure, a popular fertilizer.

Dust Mites

Carpets, comforters and feather pillows are favorite breeding grounds for microscopic dust mites, which produce an allergenic protein in their excrement. Like dander, which is allergenic because of the proteins it contains, mite-ridden dust is not an allergen unless it's in the air. Oriental rugs hanging on the wall and dusty furniture that remains undisturbed are not allergy problems. It's when a rug is walked on, releasing dander or dust mites, or when a breeze circulates dust or when a person lies down on a feather pillow or curls up under a down comforter that the proteins in dust and dander trigger allergic reactions.

Dust mites prefer warm temperatures and high humidity, conditions that are also conducive to the growth of mold, another allergen. Mold is a common problem under carpets, especially in humid climates, and it thrives on shower curtains and other bathroom surfaces. Dried flowers or plants often contain mold and anything stored in a damp basement, especially books, papers or fabric, will become musty with mold or mildew.

Water filters or distillers, air conditioners, bare floors, plastic encased mattresses, pillows made from dacron or other synthetic fibers, the scrupulous disinfecting of humidifiers and dehumidifiers, washable blankets and bedding in place of wool or down comforters, frequent dusting with a damp cloth, frequent vacuuming with special multi-layer vacuum cleaner bags that prevent the recirculation of allergens, heating system filters, window shades in place of fabric drapes, furniture without upholstery, HEPA (high-efficiency, particle-arresting) air cleaners, chemical-free cleaning products, paints and varnishes made without irritating chemicals, the removal of fuzzy stuffed toys, the professional cleaning of air ducts, lightly (rather than tightly) closed windows and doors that provide a free exchange of air instead of sealing the building, and a ban on the smoke from cigarettes, pipes, cigars, fireplaces and wood-burning stoves all reduce exposure to environmental toxins.

To reduce exposure to dust mites, some experts recommend

putting sheets, pillows and pillow cases in a hot dryer twice a week for 10 minutes, keeping stuffed animals, shaggy rugs, quilts and dolls out of the bedroom, having pets sleep away from the bedroom and rinsing the face in hot salted water. Another treatment for dust mites is tea tree oil. A dilute solution (0.8 percent tea tree oil) can be made by combining 1/2 tablespoon tea tree oil with an equal amount of rubbing alcohol or vodka (to make it water-dispersible) and 1 quart of water. Exposure to an 0.8 percent solution of tea tree oil kills 100 percent of treated dust mites within 30 minutes. Where rinsing or sponging is inconvenient, the solution can be sprayed. It can be applied to carpets through any rug shampoo appliance.

Reducing exposure reduces stress on the immune system and in some cases, that alone is all the body needs to recover and reverse the damage. See the appendix for a list of mail order companies specializing in hypoallergenic products.

House Plants Can Help

One effective air filter you don't have to send away for is the house plant. When the National Aeronautics and Space Administration (NASA) discovered in 1973 that Skylab's tightly sealed air contained over a hundred toxic chemicals, the agency began a search for solutions. Learning that Russian scientists were experimenting with live plants as air purifiers, NASA hired research scientists to explore that possibility. The researchers found that all house plants share the ability to remove contaminants from the air by pulling them into their leaves. The toxins migrate to the roots and into the soil, where they decompose. Trichlorethylene, formaldehyde and benzene, three common pollutants, were treated in sealed growth chambers by common plants such as the peace lily, lady palm and corn plant, any of which could clean the air in a small (10'-by-10') room. As the study discovered, the more house plants you have in a home or office, the more pure the air becomes. Other research has shown that the popular spider plant consumes tobacco smoke and that philodendrons and aloe vera are effective air purifiers. To help your plant collection improve the quality of indoor air, place a layer of activated carbon at the bottom of each pot before adding soil; place a drop or two of grapefruit seed extract or tea tree oil or a tablespoon of topical hydrogen peroxide in drainage dishes every week before watering to prevent the growth of mold and bacteria in standing water; keep air circulating around the plants with a low speed fan; position plants at different heights; use a variety of plants; position shade-loving plants in areas that receive little or no natural light and place sun-loving plants near windows; use at least one plant for every 100 square feet of floor space (two is better) in rooms of average height and increase the number of plants for rooms with high ceilings, in areas in which cigarettes are smoked or in homes near busy highways. Where necessary, supplement natural light with plant lights. Feed and water your green friends and they will repay you handsomely.

While mold can be a problem in greenhouses and other humid, plant-filled spaces, carefully tended house plants don't have to promote the growth of mold. The most common problem of this nature is over-watered plants that stand on carpeting. Any carpet that becomes saturated and prevented from drying out will develop serious mold and mildew infestation. Anyone concerned about potential pathogens in the potting soil can prevent its contact with the air by spreading several inches of aquarium gravel over the top of the soil, or you can spray the surface with a dilute solution of grapefruit seed extract and water. For a wealth of information on indoor gardening, see your local library and visit nurseries and plant stores.

Animal Dander

Because animal dander triggers so many adverse reactions, allergists often recommend that pets be given away. In 20 years of doctor appointments for the treatment of hay fever and asthma, I was usually told on the first office visit to get rid of my cats. Like many pet lovers who receive this prescription, I refused. None of my dozen doctors offered alternative solutions, all announced in authoritative voices that there was no way to remove the problem without removing the pets and all but one expressed annoyance and irritation at patients who refuse to cooperate.

But for every study that links pet dander to respiratory problems, others show that pet owners live longer, have happier lives, have lower stress levels and enjoy more meaningful relationships than those who don't share their lives with pets. A recent study of nursing homes showed that facilities with a resident dog have lower death rates, lower infection rates and lower staff turnover rates than those without. A study of recovering heart attack victims showed that the most significant difference between those who died within one year and those who survived was dog ownership. For many Americans, pets are members of the family. Getting rid of them, even on a doctor's orders, is as traumatic as losing a relative.

Pet dander in carpeted homes is more of a problem than in homes with bare floors, although any rug or fabric can harbor dander. The source of the problem isn't hair that the animals shed but proteins in their saliva and flakes of skin. This is why young kittens and puppies don't trigger allergic reactions; they have no old skin to shed and therefore no dander. It isn't until the age of three or four months, or even later, that pets begin to produce the allergen. This explains how someone can develop a sudden allergy to a pet that was for months a comfortable roommate.

Years ago my husband and I lived in a carpeted house and a few days after we steam-cleaned the carpets, we had a house guest who was violently allergic to animals. He kept looking at our cats and wondered why he wasn't sneezing. That's when we realized that animal dander in carpets can be washed away. We had wanted only to remove old stains but, as a bonus, we had a dander-free house.

Removing dander from rugs and carpets is only part of the solution. Washing the pets themselves is just as important. Full baths were traumatic for our elderly cats, but we found they would tolerate sponge baths. Pet stores offer products just for allergy grooming: solutions you can apply with a damp cloth or spray onto dogs, cats and birds. As an alternative, simply use plain water or an herbal tea. Don't use soap; it's too harsh, strips away protective oils and is difficult to rinse out. The secret to success in using any pet allergy product is reaching the skin. Look for dander removal products in pet supply catalogs or check with your veterinarian, groomer or pet store. If you start when a kitten is tiny, you can even convince a cat to enjoy baths. My husband's red tabby, Pumpkin, was famous for his love of water. Every week I filled a spray bottle with lukewarm chamomile tea (recommended for blonds and red-heads), sat on the floor, spread towels on my lap and soaked him to the skin while he purred and kneaded. After a vigorous drying off, he would lie in the sun until his fur was once again gorgeous, fluffy, sweet-smelling and nonallergenic.

Dog and cat owners who give their animals raw food, digestive enzymes, high-quality foods, fish oils and other nutritional supplements usually notice a rapid improvement in their animal's coat: glossy fur, healthy skin and a substantial reduction in flaking or dandruff. It makes sense to reduce the production of dander at its source.

Brush pets outdoors or wear a pollen mask while brushing inside near an air filter and follow with immediate vacuuming to reduce the accumulation of new dander. Remember that cat dander is so light that most vacuum cleaners merely redistribute it; if you're serious about controlling dander and dust mites, you need a vacuum cleaner equipped with special high-filtration bags. For best results, use carpet steam-cleaning equipment as well.

Of course, in some cases radical measures are necessary. Some people have had to find new homes for their pets when other measures failed to prevent life-threatening asthma attacks in themselves or their children. The strategies described here don't work for everyone but what many pet owners don't realize is that these strategies exist at all. I believe they're worth trying before dogs and cats are banished from any caring home.

THE IMPORTANCE OF DIET

External strategies work well to reduce the factors that trigger allergies, asthma and other breathing problems, but none of them cure the illness. Neither do standard prescription drugs, for their function is to suppress symptoms, not correct causes.

In addition to using the tactics described above, you can treat respiratory illness from the inside out, repairing and improving the immune system so that everyday exposure to low levels of environmental toxins doesn't wreak havoc on the lungs. This same approach helps prevent colds, flu, bronchitis, asthma attacks, hay fever symptoms and sinus congestion. In fact, many experts claim that the true cause of hay fever isn't pollen or dust mites or animal dander at all; it's the human body that interprets these substances as dangerous intruders and activates the immune system to repel them. Correcting this misinterpretation can be done with herbs and diet.

How to Test For Food Sensitivities

Most Americans eat a monotonous diet of wheat, dairy products, refined salt, caffeine beverages, carbonated beverages containing high-fructose corn syrup, meat, chicken and eggs. These foods may be arranged in different ways so it seems as though we're eating a variety of foods, but a breakfast of pancakes or waffles or muffins is the same as a cheeseburger lunch or a pizza dinner. These meals are different combinations of refined wheat flour and milk or cheese.

Food choices are of special interest to health professionals who treat respiratory problems because these illnesses are so often linked to food sensitivities, and food sensitivities often result from a monotonous diet.

Physicians who study food sensitivities say the most common offenders are milk and wheat, followed by eggs, chocolate, corn, citrus fruit, beans, peas, tomatoes, nuts, fish, preservatives, cola beverages and food additives. If you eat a food often enough, especially if your body is already stressed by environmental factors or inefficient digestion, you can develop an intolerance to it.

A simple way to treat allergies, asthma, bronchitis, chronic sinus congestion, chronic cough, hay fever, chronic ear infections in adults or children and similar afflictions is to avoid all milk products (milk, cream, ice cream, ice milk, cheese, cottage cheese, yogurt, frozen yogurt, cream cheese, sour cream and foods containing nonfat milk solids) and all wheat products (breads, crackers, pastries, pasta, pretzels) for a month. In many cases, the condition improves quickly. I can recommend this strategy from experience, for I have had severe hay fever symptoms from childhood, diagnosed by blood tests as allergies to animal dander, pollens, dust mites and grasses. Yet I live comfortably with dogs and cats and avoid hay fever symptoms by avoiding wheat and dairy. If I eat cheese, yogurt or products containing milk solids, especially in combination with wheat bread or pasta, I'm sneezing within an hour. As one allergist explained, eating those foods puts sufficient stress on my immune system so that exposure to animal dander, dust mites or pollen results in a full-blown allergy attack. By the simple strategy of avoiding certain foods, I avoid hay fever symptoms.

There is much debate and confusion over the term "food allergy." To orthodox physicians, an allergic reaction is immediate and dramatic, like anaphylactic shock, which can be fatal, or a sudden eruption of hives. The term "food sensitivity" was coined to describe more subtle reactions that are still debilitating.

Although there are blood tests and patch tests designed to detect food allergies and sensitivities, you can conduct your own effective test at home with pencil in hand. Keep a notebook of everything you eat, when you eat it, how your body responds and how you feel. Sometimes this simple exercise will bring to light an obvious connection between cause and symptom.

A more serious test is the four-day rotation diet. Because it takes four days for the body to remove all traces of the foods you consume, this system schedules four days of menus according to related food groups. On day one, for example, you might eat wheat, then no wheat at all on days two, three and four.

Other approaches to allergy and food sensitivity testing are applied kinesiology, a form of muscle testing, and pulse diagnosis, a simple procedure discovered 50 years ago by Arthur M. Coca, M.D., author of *The Pulse Test*. Coca discovered that when you eat a food that agrees with you, your pulse rate remains stable. If you eat one that doesn't, it increases.

In order to take the pulse test accurately, you must stop smoking for the duration of the test and be free of conditions that might disrupt your pulse, such as fighting off a cold or being sunburned.

Count your pulse for 60 seconds just after waking in the morning and just before going to bed at night. In addition, take it just before each meal and again 30 minutes, 60 minutes and 90 minutes after the meal ends. Always take your pulse sitting up, except when you first wake.

Keep a food journal for two or three days, noting everything you eat at each meal and the day's pulse rates. Some connections may be obvious at once. If your pulse jumps from 65 beats per minute just before breakfast to 85 beats per minute after, something in the French toast may not agree with you. One woman discovered that her pulse raced every morning, just after she got out of bed. After three days of record keeping, she realized that the problem was her toothpaste. When she changed brands, her chronic migraine headaches disappeared.

You can use the pulse test to check individual foods and narrow your findings to a single offender. Dr. Coca recommended checking the pulse at half-hour intervals, but my experiments suggest that most reactions are apparent within five minutes.

Learning your food sensitivities is one thing; working around them is something else, especially if your strongest reactions are to wheat and dairy products. Wheat and milk are everywhere. Your health food store is an important source of cookbooks, nonwheat flours, dairy-free ice creams and cheeses, nonwheat pastas and milk substitutes. No, these foods don't taste like the real thing, but if you can't have the real thing, they're worth trying. Because of increased demand and competition, the substitute foods market is still improving, and it's growing fast. Even supermarkets are beginning to carry substitute products. Shopping for restricted diets is still a challenge, but it's not the lonely task it was 20 years ago.

Eat More Raw Food

Raw foods contain nutrients and enzymes that are destroyed by cooking. The human digestive tract is designed to process a diet consisting of a wide variety of foods, much of it raw and unprocessed.

Juice fasting, which is a modified type of fast consisting of only freshly made juices and water or tea, lets the body rest and recuperate. Several effective therapies for not only respiratory problems but serious diseases such as cancer are based on fresh juices. A short-term juice fast, lasting a few days or a week, can bring relief from many respiratory symptoms.

Water-only fasts are controversial for medical reasons, but juice fasting provides more nutrients and less exposure to common allergens than the normal American diet. Health claims made for juice therapies on late-night television may be exaggerated, but for the person fighting chronic hay fever, asthma or other respiratory problems, several days of drinking freshly made juices may bring a welcome respite from symptoms. Instead of resuming your normal diet all at once, introduce foods one at a time and monitor your reaction. Every person's response to foods and food groups is unique, and this is a simple way to test foods and their effects on the body.

Experts on juice fasting recommend avoiding the juice of any fruit or vegetable you may be allergic or sensitive to, diluting juices with high sugar content, such as carrot or beet juice, with low sugar juices, such as celery; diluting fruit juices with an equal amount of water; and avoiding juice fasting if you are pregnant or lactating. Medical supervision is recommended for diabetics and others with serious illnesses.

Improve Your Digestion

Many people with hay fever allergies suffer from candidiasis, the overgrowth of the yeast/fungus *Candida albicans* in the digestive tract. This microorganism occurs naturally in the human body, but its overgrowth is the cause of yeast infections, and it disrupts normal digestion. Candidiasis is often triggered by antibiotics, as these drugs kill the beneficial bacteria that normally keep Candida in check. Candida thrives on sugars and refined carbohydrates, which is why it's so widespread in America. Orthodox therapy includes dietary restrictions (no sugars, carbohydrates, fruits, alcohol or fermented foods) and the use of antifungal drugs. Holistic therapy combines dietary restrictions with such herbal antifungal agents as pau d'arco tea (also called Taheebo) and grapefruit seed or citrus seed extract.

The most important part of Candida therapy is the reestablishment of normal intestinal flora, the "friendly" bacteria that promote complete digestion and prevent the overgrowth of Candida. One approach is to eat yogurt, which contains acidophilus and similar bacteria; another is to take acidophilus supplements, which are widely sold in health food stores. For those who are unable to digest cow's milk, or who have an adverse reaction to it, soy yogurts are available, or you can make your own at home from soy milk and acidophilus or yogurt starter. In addition to supplementing the diet with acidophilus, bifidus and related bacteria, consider taking a small amount of Swedish bitters or any fresh bitter-tasting herb such as dandelion leaves just before eating. Bitter tastes stimulate the production and secretion of important digestive fluids, such as bile.

With age, the body's production of digestive enzymes and digestive secretions decreases, creating a variety of health complications. Indigestion is sometimes a symptom of insufficient hydrochloric acid, not an excess, so taking antacid tablets after eating may contribute to the problem rather than prevent it. Dozens of digestive enzyme products, many containing hydrochloric acid, are available in drugstores and health food stores. A nutritionally oriented physician or health care professional can help you determine exactly what type of supplement will be most helpful in improving your digestion.

Avoid Sulfites and Other Additives

People with asthma or allergies may find their symptoms alleviated by the simple strategy of avoiding chemical preservatives and artificial coloring. Sulfur dioxide, sodium bisulfite and sulfites are used to prevent dryness, stiffening and discoloration in dried fruits, frozen potatoes, shrimp, avocado dips, salads, vegetables, wine, beer and other foods. According to Michael Murray, N.D., and Joseph Pizzorno, N.D., in their *Encyclopedia of Natural Medicine,* a restaurant customer can easily ingest up to 100 mg of metabisulphite in a single meal. Asthma attacks can be triggered by exposure to sulfites, tartrazine (an orange food dye) and benzoates (preservatives), and at least four deaths caused by sulfites have been reported to the Food and Drug Administration. Always check labels for additives and, in general, try to avoid processed foods that contain chemicals.

How can you tell if the food in a restaurant or supermarket has been treated with sulfites? If the management displays a sign claiming "no sulfites," it's probably true. In 1986, the FDA made the use of sulfites on fresh produce illegal, so salad bars are less a hazard than they used to be. Still, prepared foods may contain sulfites and it's best to be sure. The demand for a simple way of determining sulfite content inspired the development of sulfite test strips, which can be dipped into any food. The strips turn red, revealing the presence of sulfites, or green, showing that the food is sulfite-free.

Consider Nutritional Supplements

Vitamins and minerals have been used to treat illnesses other than obvious nutritional deficiencies for over 70 years.

Jonathan Wright, M.D., treated a child who suffered from chronic nasal congestion and who had been repeatedly admitted to hospital emergency rooms for wheezing. Antihistamine medication failed to improve his condition. Wright diagnosed the boy's problem as an inability to digest and absorb nutrients, and he prescribed vitamin B12 injections, digestive supplements, magnesium and other minerals. The patient's health improved quickly and he has had no further wheezing attacks.

Not all of the dosages used in orthomolecular medicine are in the megavitamin category, but some are dramatic multiples of the standard daily recommendations. To reduce hay fever or asthma symptoms, a physician might recommend 5 to 20 grams of powdered ascorbic acid (vitamin C) to be taken in small doses with water over a 24-hour period. A mild cold may be prevented by taking 30 to 60 grams, influenza with 100 to 150 grams and viral pneumonia with dosages up to 200 grams in 24 hours. Considering that a 500 mg tablet (1/2 gram) is considered a high dose of vitamin C, these recommendations are unusual and they should not be taken without supervision. This treatment for the prevention of an acute infection lasts for several days or until all symptoms disappear. The dosage remains high until the body indicates its vitamin C saturation point by developing loose bowels, a signal to reduce the amount. Many orthomolecular physicians have found that taking vitamin C to bowel tolerance (the diarrhea point) effectively treats colds, flu, infections, allergies, burns, viral pneumonia and autoimmune disorders.

In general, those with respiratory infections or illnesses benefit from the daily use of a well-balanced multiple vitamin and mineral supplement and additional trace minerals.

Breastfeed Your Baby

The evidence for this health benefit is overwhelming. Breastfeeding protects children from all kinds of respiratory infections, ear infections, allergies and asthma. Many pediatricians trace their patients' allergies and ear infections to exposure to cow's milk in infant formulas. If a breastfed baby experiences colic or allergic symptoms, it is often because the mother ate something that disagreed with her own physiology as well as her baby's.

In fact, the mother's diet is the most important factor in breastfeeding. According to pediatrician Lendon Smith, an expert on nutrition and the author of several books on children's health, milk, soy, corn, wheat and eggs are frequent offenders, while a baby's colic can be caused by the mother eating garlic, onion, beans or cabbage. Dr. Smith recommends that nursing mothers avoid these foods.

Saying that a nursing mother should avoid dairy products goes against everything we are taught by physicians and the dairy industry's ad campaigns, but stop and think. Do you really need milk to produce milk? Cows don't drink milk and neither do other milk-producing animals. Millions of women around the world drink no milk at all and nurse their babies successfully. Only in the U.S., Canada and parts of Europe do people assume that successful nursing requires a diet rich in dairy products.

If the indirect consumption of dairy products creates problems for infants, their direct consumption creates more. Raw, unpasteurized, unhomogenized cow's milk is the ideal food for baby calves. Pasteurized, homogenized cow's milk is far from ideal for calves and even farther from ideal for human babies. According to Dr. Smith, cow's milk formulas such as SMA, Similac and Enfamil may precipitate colic, diarrhea, rashes, ear infections, asthma and other conditions in up to 50 percent of the infants who drink them.

Long-term nursing has been shown to provide the maximum lifelong health benefits, but nursing remains unfashionable in the U.S. and new mothers are often pressured to switch from breast to bottle.

Be Inspired — or else.

SUPPORT THERAPIES FOR ALL RESPIRATORY CONDITIONS

Drink More Water

In his book, *Your Body's Many Cries for Water*, F. Batmanghelidj, M.D., explained that many symptoms of major and minor illnesses are caused not by disease but by dehydration. "You are not sick," he wrote, "you are thirsty!" *Your Body's Many Cries for Water* is widely recommended by medical doctors and health care professionals because it offers a simple, inexpensive, often dramatically effective cure for indigestion, intestinal problems, rheumatoid arthritis pain, stress, depression, high blood pressure, overweight, asthma, allergies and other disorders.

Dr. Batmanghelidj's therapy could not be simpler. At

the first sign of symptoms, drink an 8-ounce glass of water. After 15 to 20 minutes, drink another. Continue drinking plain water throughout the day and do so every day so that the body is properly hydrated. In adults, this may be a gallon of water daily. Tea, coffee, cola beverages, soft drinks and juices don't count; what matters is plain water. In addition, Dr. Batmanghelidj recommends a small amount of unrefined sea salt daily, especially in cases of asthma, which he believes is not a disease but rather a physiological adaptation of the body to dehydration and an insufficiency of salt. Salt is a natural decongestant. "A pinch of salt on the tongue after drinking water fools the brain into thinking a lot of salt has arrived in the body," he wrote. "It is then that the brain begins to relax the bronchioles. People with asthma should slightly increase their salt intake."

No discussion of water would be complete without a caution regarding American tap water, which has received much negative publicity in recent years. Concerns over water safety have made bottled spring water a growth industry along with home water filters and distillers. Whatever you can do to improve the quality of the water you drink will help improve your health.

Use Unrefined Salt

Americans are so used to hearing physicians' warnings against salt that Dr. Batmanghelidj's advice to increase salt consumption sounds strange. But he's right. While refined table salt causes serious problems, natural salt improves every body function.

All popular brands of table salt have been bleached, then treated with stabilizing agents and dehydrating chemicals. Whether coarse or finely ground, this salt is between 98 and 99 percent pure sodium chloride (NaCl), and it was dried at temperatures high enough to change its crystalline structure. Its structural changes, nutrient stripping and added chemicals make table salt difficult for the body to assimilate, contributing to electrolyte imbalances, trace mineral deficiencies, digestive problems, fluid retention and high blood pressure. The sodium content of nearly every processed food derives from refined salt.

Unfortunately, nearly all brands of sea salt have been refined. Most sea salt is 98 to 99 percent pure sodium chloride and, like table salt, it contains no trace minerals, only the residue of processing chemicals. Let appearance and flavor guide you. If a salt is bright white (unrefined rock salt or mined salt is beige in color, unrefined sea salt is gray), if it is iodized (iodine added), if its crystals are large like kosher salt prior to grinding, if it pours easily in humid conditions and if it has the sharp, familiar taste of table salt, it's best avoided.

Natural salt is of special interest to herbalists. Traditionally, herbal teas were served salted to enhance the healing properties of "simples" and blends. A pinch of unrefined salt added to a glass of water or pot of tea helps balance the body's electrolytes and provides trace minerals often lacking in the food we eat. For a more effective alternative to commercial sports beverages, add a pinch of unrefined sea salt to water and a splash of juice for flavor.

Remember Dr. Batmanghelidj's advice to hold a pinch of salt on the tongue after drinking water for relief from respiratory congestion and to increase salt consumption in general if you suffer from asthma or allergies.

Stop Smoking

For many Americans, this is easier said than done. Smoking is a chemical addiction that those who don't smoke find incomprehensible. It takes more than will power, resolutions, good intentions, pleas from friends and relatives, public ordinances, medical problems and high cigarette prices to stop smoking.

If you have a respiratory illness, smoking will make it worse. If you live with someone who does, secondhand smoke will do the same. People still argue about the links between smoking and heart disease or breast cancer, but the links between smoking and emphysema, asthma, lung cancer and other respiratory problems are well-documented. Chewing tobacco, which has gained in popularity in recent years, has its own adverse side effects, including cancers of the mouth and throat.

Of all the approaches to quitting, and there are many, two of the most effective may be acupuncture and orthomolecular medicine. Acupuncture has an impressive record in treating all kinds of addictions, not just smoking, as does orthomolecular medicine, which treats illness with nutritional supplements.

In the Winter 1993 issue of *The Herb Quarterly,* herbalist Elizabeth Phillips reviewed plants that help smokers quit. "These herbs will regulate a smoker's mood (no more irritability)," she wrote, "and the accompanying urge to overeat as nicotine intake stops, and they will cleanse the system of nicotine and the lungs of tar sediment. And they will do all that simply, easily and safely."

The herbs in Phillips's program are the sedative herbs valerian root, chamomile and skullcap; licorice root and comfrey, which reduce the symptoms of drug withdrawal; black cohosh, burdock root and red clover for blood cleansing; slippery elm bark and fenugreek, which help remove mucus from the lungs; catnip, magnolia and peppermint, which aid the smoker in quitting; and echinacea to support the immune system. These herbs are alternated during the program so you use slightly different combinations every day.

To brew each tea, bring 1/2 cup water to a boil in a small, pan (the recipes are for 4-ounce teacups), add the required amount of dry herbs, cover and let stand for 10 minutes. Strain and serve.

Phillips advised starting the day with a 4-ounce cup of tea made with 1/2 teaspoon each of chamomile (or scullcap) and

valerian root. At mid-morning, mix 1/2 teaspoon licorice root
with 1/2 teaspoon comfrey leaf. At noon, brew 1/2 teaspoon
black cohosh with 1/2 teaspoon burdock root or red clover.
In the early afternoon, combine 1/2 teaspoon slippery elm
bark with 1/2 teaspoon fenugreek. Discontinue this tea when
you stop coughing up mucus. In the late afternoon, mix 1/2
teaspoon magnolia with 1/2 teaspoon peppermint or catnip.
Just before dinner, brew a cup of echinacea tea using 1 teaspoon echinacea leaf. Sweeten any of these teas with honey
or add a pinch of the herb stevia, a popular alternative to
sugar. In addition, Phillips recommended taking 500 mg of
vitamin C, a vitamin E capsule and one tablet of goldenseal
root daily, although goldenseal, like untreated licorice root,
is not recommended for those with heart disease.

Since Phillips's article was published, comfrey has been
removed from many health food stores because of its alleged
toxicity (see page 65). I would not hesitate to take the small
amount of comfrey called for here, but you should study the
evidence and make your own decision. If you decide not to
use comfrey, substitute burdock root or red clover.

In addition to the herbs recommended above, here are
three that can be real friends to anyone who is trying to quit
smoking. The first is lobelia or Indian tobacco; the second
is calamus root. Because both of these herbs come with FDA
warnings, please read their descriptions carefully before
using. The third helpful herb is oat grass or oatstraw, a tonic
for the nerves.

It is easy to become discouraged if you try to quit smoking
and fail. But there are so many approaches to this project
that if you really want to stop, you will find one that works.

RESPIRATORY CONDITIONS

Allergies and Hay Fever

The word "allergy" did not exist in Shakespeare's time or even a hundred years ago. It's a modern term for a modern illness—or, more accurately, an assortment of illnesses. Allergy is a catchall word for a variety of reactions made by the body when it detects something foreign. The offending substances may be foods, animal dander, house dust, pollens, mold, smoke, air pollution, medicines or chemicals. The ability of the immune system to identify individual substances and react to them is crucial, but overreaction creates uncomfortable symptoms such as sneezing, sinus congestion, itching or watery eyes, headaches, indigestion, skin rashes, hives and other symptoms.

At any time of year, it can be hard to tell the difference between allergies and cold symptoms. Either can produce sneezes, a runny nose, nasal congestion, an itchy throat and irritated cough. If a "cold" lasts for several weeks, and if your symptoms seem more severe in certain locations (less intense outdoors in winter, for example, and worse in certain rooms or buildings), it's probably hay fever.

According to allergy researchers, indoor or year-round allergies are almost always due to three sources of irritation:

the droppings of microscopic dust mites that live in house dust, mold spores and animal dander. In many households, the causes may also include cockroach parts, rodent urine or the smoke from a wood-burning stove or fireplace. All of these irritants are associated with asthma as well. See pages 5 to 9 (pet dander, dust mites) for tips on reducing exposure to pet dander and dust mites.

The orthodox treatment of allergies includes the use of decongestants, antihistamines and steroid drugs. Some allergists specialize in desensitization shots, in which small quantities of allergenic substances are injected into the body over a period of time. Desensitization therapy for bee stings and other insect venoms is generally effective, according to Philip S. Norman in his 1980 overview of immunotherapy published in the *Journal of Allergy and Clinical Immunology,* while scientific studies on the effectiveness of desensitization to pollen, molds, house dust and animal danders are "generally inconclusive or lacking."

The link between diet and allergies is important, and anyone hoping to relieve hay fever symptoms and allergic reactions to dust mites, pet dander and other common irritants will do well to explore food sensitivities.

Honey and Bee Pollen. Honey contains pollen, and some hay fever sufferers swear by honey from local bees. Their strategy is to eat comb honey or raw, unheated, unrefined, unfiltered honey from local bees in three-day cycles for several weeks before hay fever season. This exposure acts like a vaccination and makes the local pollens less irritating.

Bee pollen is a popular food supplement, but I have misgivings about recommending it to those who have hay fever. Some seriously adverse reactions have been reported among people with severe allergies who took bee pollen, probably because the dose is so concentrated compared to what you would ingest in a spoonful of honey. A better approach is to start with a single grain per day three to four months before hay fever season and slowly increase the dosage, adding one grain every three days. Discontinue if you experience any adverse symptoms, such as sinus congestion, throat irritation, fatigue, headaches, nausea, abdominal pain, diarrhea, itchy skin or memory problems, all of which may occur when someone allergic to pollen takes bee pollen capsules daily for several weeks. The physician who reported these symptoms noted that bee pollen capsules, despite manufacturer's claims, do not contain only pollen from plants that are pollinated by bees but also contain allergenic airborne pollens such as ragweed.

For best results, never experiment with more than a single grain of bee pollen or a tiny amount of raw honey if you are trying this approach for the first time. Of course, for honey "vaccinations" to work, the raw honey or bee pollen must come from local hives and contain local pollens.

Homeopathy. The bee pollen approach to hay fever resembles homeopathy, for both strategies introduce small amounts of allergenic substances in hopes that the body will respond and overcome the illness. The difference is in the dosage. Homeopathic hay fever preparations are extremely dilute solutions of the yeasts, molds, grasses, tree pollens, fungi, animal dander, dust mites and other airborne allergens that typically cause reactions. Respiratory illnesses such as hay fever are among the conditions homeopathy is best known for treating.

A similar strategy is used by people who take **ragweed** tincture in the spring and early summer, before this plant flowers. The Heritage Store in Virginia sells products recommended by Edgar Cayce, the American psychic whose well documented medical insights cured thousands during the 1930s and '40s. Edgar Cayce recommended ragweed to over a hundred individuals as a liver tonic and nonhabit-forming laxative and prescribed it to help desensitize pollen-sensitive systems when taken ahead of pollen season. Users have reported relief from other allergies after taking ragweed tincture for several weeks.

The Heritage Store's product contains only ragweed and grain alcohol. Inspired when I read this at the peak of ragweed season as I was sneezing my head off, I gathered blossoms from the inconspicuous common ragweed (*Artemesia artemisifolia*) and the tree-tall great or giant ragweed (*A. trifida*), covered the pollen-rich flowers with vodka and made my own tincture. The following spring I began taking half a dropperful daily. All through ragweed season, which lasts to the end of October, I continued the ragweed experiment and seldom sneezed, even when pollen counts hit record highs.

Herbs That Can Help. If you don't have high blood pressure, the Chinese herb **Ma huang** (*ephedra vulgaris*) may be helpful. The active ingredient in most commercial allergy preparations made from herbs, Ma huang or Chinese ephedra is a powerful decongestant. It clears bronchial passageways, dries sinuses, helps relieve sneezing and makes breathing easier. It also speeds the pulse, raises blood pressure, makes it difficult to relax and feels like caffeine. The more you take, the more dramatic these side effects, so start with a small amount, don't take Ma huang in the evening (it may keep you awake) and, if brewing a tea with this herb, make a weak infusion to start.

Nettle (*Urtica dioica*) may sting when you touch it, but nettle tea soothes the system. In "A Randomized Double-Blind Study of Freeze-Dried *Urtica dioica* in the Treatment of Allergic Rhinitis," published in the journal *Planta Medica* (February 1990), P. Mittman reported significant hay fever relief from capsules containing freeze-dried nettle. The therapy had few side effects and improvement came within a week for those who found the treatment effective. Andrew Weil, M.D., author of *Spontaneous Healing,* controls his own hay fever with this therapy. Nettle tea and fresh nettle juice are used in Europe for a variety of conditions, including several respiratory problems.

Echinacea and **goldenseal** are a favorite combination for hay fever therapy. In fact, many herbalists consider goldenseal the most effective botanical treatment for acute sinus infections because it fights bacteria and viruses while soothing mucous membranes. Both herbs support the immune system. Teas and tinctures made with **red clover, sage, burdock root** or **licorice root** are often recommended for hay fever prevention and treatment and all have much to recommend them.

Gail Ulrich, herbalist and director of the Blazing Star Herbal School recommends an infusion of dried **mullein** leaf (2 tablespoons or 1 ounce by volume of the dried herb per quart of boiling water) steeped 2 to 4 hours and given in ½ cup doses 4 times daily for 6 weeks to eliminate allergies to pet dander and relieve other allergy symptoms.

Rosemary Gladstar has an unusual recipe for **garlic-ginger** syrup that helps prevent allergies and hay fevers. See page 41 for the recipe.

Other Approaches. The food supplement quercetin, a bioflavonoid, has been shown to relieve or prevent hay fever and allergy symptoms, and the nutritional support offered by vitamin/mineral supplements is important as well. Vitamin C is a natural antihistamine, and large doses during hay fever season may bring relief. Orothomolecular physicians recommend as much as 5 to 20 grams of vitamin C taken in 4 to 8 doses over 24 hours for this condition.

Salt is another decongestant. To treat hay fever symptoms, drink an 8-ounce glass of water followed by a pinch of salt on the tongue every 15 to 30 minutes until symptoms subside. The same strategy will work for asthma.

Mechanical aids make a difference, too. Breathe Right nasal strips are a familiar sight in professional football games, where players use them to keep nasal passages clear when plastic mouth guards interfere with normal respiration. Advertised as a drug-free way to relieve snoring as well as nasal congestion due to allergies, colds and deviated septums, these strips are sold in drugstores and in health supply catalogs.

A simple way to break the hay fever cycle without drugs is to go on a week-long cleansing juice fast, drinking only

water and freshly prepared raw fruit and vegetable juices and
eating no solid food at all. If you're like most hay fever
sufferers, your sneezing symptoms will diminish or disappear, suggesting a link to food sensitivities.

Asthma

A full-blown asthma attack is a nightmare: you can't catch
your breath. Add coughing, rattly wheezing, a choking sensation and the light-headed feeling that accompanies a lack of
oxygen and you get the idea. Asthma is worse than inconvenient; it can be fatal. In the United States, asthma has become
an epidemic, especially among children. Orthodox physicians
treat it with steroids, antihistamines, bronchiole dilators and
other drugs, all of which have adverse side effects and none
of which address asthma's cause.

"Extrinsic" or "atopic" asthma is related to allergies and
brings a characteristic increase in the blood serum immuno-
globulin IgE. "Intrinsic" asthma does not involve allergies;
it is triggered by chemicals, exposure to cold air or water, active
physical exercise, infection or emotional upset. Recent research
by Michael Burr at the Center for Applied Public Health Medicine in Cardiff, Wales, found that industrial pollution with sulfur
dioxide and smoke does not cause asthma but appears to increase its severity. The study blamed diesel exhaust fumes and
ozone for increasing the allergic effects of inhaled allergens and
noted a rise in asthma cases in areas with decreasing industrial
pollution but increasing automobile traffic. Until hydrogen re-
places petroleum as a fuel, large cities and busy roads will
make life more difficult for asthma patients.

The Allergic Connection. No matter what conditions trigger an asthma attack, naturopathic physicians believe that asthma's underlying causes are food sensitivities
or food allergies, insufficient hydrochloric acid (even among
children), leading to incomplete digestion, and exposure to

food additives and other chemicals that overburden the immune system, causing it to malfunction. Diets that eliminate common allergens have been effective in treating asthmatic adults and children. Double-blind food challenges in children have shown that sensitivities resulting in immediate symptoms are most likely to involve eggs, fish, shellfish, nuts and peanuts, while those resulting in the delayed onset of symptoms are most likely to involve milk, chocolate, wheat, citrus fruits and food coloring. Of course, every person is different, and the best way to tell what foods may be triggering your or your child's symptoms is to keep a food diary, experiment with food groups and rotation diets, try applied kinesiology's muscle testing or see a health care professional who specializes in nutrition.

In someone whose production of hydrochloric acid is insufficient for complete digestion, discovering the causes of food allergies and eliminating them is only part of the solution, for unless the low stomach acid is corrected, new food sensitivities will develop as new foods replace old ones. According to Jonathan Wright, M.D., one of the diseases associated with low stomach acid is childhood asthma. This deficiency is easy to diagnose and the cure is inexpensive. Digestive supplements containing hydrochloric acid are sold in health food stores.

In 1993, *The Journal of Allergy and Clinical Immunology* reported on a respiratory technologist who developed occupational asthma after being exposed to sterilizing agents in her work. Whenever she cleaned bronchoscopes, her asthma worsened.

The sterilizing agent glutaraldehyde may be unusual, but most American homes have their own share of asthma-aggravating allergens. In 1993 *The American Journal of Epidemiology* reported on a study of 457 asthmatic Canadian children ages 3 to 4, which compared them to 457 control subjects. Independent risk factors for asthma included heavy smoking by the mother, the use of a humidifier in the child's room and an electric heating system in the house. Less important but still significant were the presence of other smokers in the home, a history of pneumonia, the absence of breastfeeding and a family history of asthma. Other studies have shown that smoke from a fireplace or wood stove can aggravate asthma, as can a host of common household cleansers, paints, paint thinners, perfumes and some types of incense.

The problem with humidifiers, which are supposed to help relieve respiratory congestion, is that they are breeding grounds for molds, bacteria and other germs. To prevent these problems, add liquid **grapefruit seed extract** to your humidifier's water reservoir. Grapefruit seed or citrus seed extract, which kills viruses, bacteria, yeasts, molds, parasites and other pathogens on contact even when greatly diluted, is sold in health food stores. **Tea tree oil** has similar properties, in addition to a sinus-clearing antiseptic fragrance reminiscent of eucalyptus oil and turpentine. In fact, some people relieve sinus congestion by placing a drop on the upper lip, just under the nose, at bedtime. Unlike liquid grapefruit seed extract, tea tree oil is not water-soluble, so for best results, dissolve a teaspoon of tea tree oil with an equal or larger amount of vodka or other alcohol before mixing it with water. To disinfect a humidifier that is used daily, add 1/8 teaspoon of liquid grapefruit seed extract or tea tree oil/vodka solution to the water reservoir once a week, and add several drops of either solution to the reservoir daily. For more about these two products, see my booklet, *Nature's Antiseptics: Tea Tree Oil and Grapefruit Seed Extract.*

A 1984 study in the *New England Journal of Medicine* found that almost one out of every five people with asthma or allergies experienced symptoms when their car's air conditioner was turned on. Prem Kumar, M.D., a professor of medicine at the Louisiana State University Medical Center, discovered that the culprit was mold. He found a variety of molds in the circulating air of 22 of the 25 patients' cars he studied. Large quantities of mold can be emitted from auto air conditioners, especially in a short, heavily concentrated burst soon after the air conditioner is turned on. This condition, most prevalent in warm, humid climates, usually generates an unpleasant odor. In response, auto makers developed an "air conditioning odor treatment" that eliminates and prevents the growth of molds, yeast, bacteria and viruses in air conditioners. Check with your dealer or service center for solutions to the car air conditioning problem.

One overlooked producer of household allergens is the cockroach. The December 1993 medical journal *Insights in Allergy* published an extensive review of the role of cockroach allergens and the incidence of asthma, concluding, "It is possible that 20 percent to 30 percent of hospital admissions associated with indoor allergens in urban areas could be attributable to cockroach sensitization. Patients who have asthma caused by indoor allergens should be routinely evaluated for cockroach sensitivity."

A similar source of irritation is the dust mite. The January 1994 *Journal of Allergy and Clinical Immunology* reviewed 22 patients whose asthma symptoms worsened in one building and disappeared in another. Researchers measured a higher level of dust mite in the first building. Environmental control is one of the most overlooked means of reducing any allergic symptom, especially asthma. For specific dust mite prevention strategies, see pages 5 and 6.

Medical research has linked asthma to a variety of food additives. The May 1993 edition of the medical journal *Canadian Family Physician* concluded that the most prevalent type of additives that induce problems are sulfites and monosodium glutamate. "Sulfites have been known to cause asthma, anaphylaxis, abdominal pain, hives, seizures, and even death," said the report. "Monosodium glutamate [a flavor enhancer] is most noted in Chinese Restaurant Syndrome and can cause immediate or late triggering of asthma. Tartrazine [an orange food coloring] can cause asthma and hives. Tartrazine is found in jams, some butter, candies, cakes and tablets."

A Japanese physician at the National Children's Hospital in Tokyo has discovered that cold water may cure some asthmas. As David Williams, M.D. reported in the May 1994 edition of his newsletter *Alternatives,* Dr. Toshio Katsunuma described an ongoing study involving 25 asthmatic children ages 4 to 20. Each child was given a cold shower every day in which 20 buckets of 59 degree Fahrenheit water were poured over the child for one minute. Twenty other patients received a warmer shower, in which the water was 86 degrees F. There was no change in this group, but all those who took cold showers required less asthma medication and some were able to discontinue medication altogether. None of the cold water treatments triggered an asthma attack. As Dr. Williams remarked, "I doubt there's a kid anywhere who wouldn't rather take a one-minute cold shower every morning than put up with the side effects and social stigma of asthma medication and inhalers."

Because exposure to cold water can trigger intrinsic asthma attacks, this approach is the opposite of what most American physicians would recommend. But a cold water shower, approached cautiously and in the absence of any history of asthma triggered by exposure to cold air or water, is a simple experiment.

Supplements. For many asthma sufferers, relief comes from nutrition. In addition to vitamins and mineral supplements that repair tissues and boost immunity, many physicians recommend bioflavonids, quercetin, bromelin and coenzyme Q10, all of which may help reduce the frequency and severity of asthma attacks. Vitamins A, B complex, C and E are considered most important, along with magnesium, selenium, and beta carotene.

In fact, vitamin C may be more significant than previously realized. In 1995 *The American Journal of Clinical Nutrition* published a report showing that a diet low in vitamin C is a risk factor for asthma, particularly in environments containing tobacco smoke and similar oxidants. According to this article, 7 of 11 studies on vitamin C have shown significant improvement in respiratory measurement within two hours after the patients took 1 to 2 grams of vitamin C. These studies are the first to show such a positive correlation and the first to use large doses of the vitamin. Previous trials using 500 mg or less were less conclusive.

Vitamin C has been shown to have antihistamine properties; it inhibits experimentally induced bronchial constriction in normal and asthmatic subjects, and in double-blind controlled studies, doses of 1 gram per day have been shown to be an effective, though not curative, preventive measure for some patients with bronchial asthma.

Herbs That Can Help. Proponents of raw food diets claim that the elimination of most cooked or processed foods and the substitution of fresh, raw fruits and vegetables can cure asthma or at least reduce its most severe symptoms. Green beverages such as freshly pressed wheat grass or barley juice and the supplementation of green or blue-green algae and similar foods may also bring relief.

Herbs have a vital place in asthma therapy. The most frequently prescribed include **echinacea, horsetail, juniper berries, licorice root, mullein** and **Ma huang. Lobelia** tincture may be helpful during asthma attacks, as it relaxes bronchial muscles. **Ginkgo,** which contains the active ingredient ginkgolide B, has shown good results in many studies.

The Chinese herb **Ma huang** (*Ephedra vulgaris*) has been used to treat asthma for more than 5,000 years. It stimulates the sympathetic nervous system and relieves bronchial spasms, making it among the most widely used herbal asthma medications. However, its common side effects include rapid pulse, increased blood pressure, nervousness and irritability. These can be reduced by taking the herb in small doses several times a day in combination with calming herbs.

According to the herbalist Christopher Hobbes in the September 1992 issue of *Natural Healing,* teas or extracts of the expectorant herbs **grindelia** and **yerba santa** are best for asthma accompanied by a heavy white sputum, while the moisturizing herbs **coltsfoot, marshmallow root, mullein** and **licorice** are better for dry types of asthma.

Rosemary Gladstar's recipe for **garlic-ginger** syrup, which treats both allergies and asthma, appears on page xx.

A New York teacher of herbal medicine, Robin Bennett has seen asthma attacks interrupted by lighting dry **mullein leaves**, blowing the flame out and inhaling the smoke. Someone assisting can hold a fireproof container (such as an ashtray) of smoking leaves within a few inches of the person's face until normal breathing resumes (about 30 to 60 seconds). This simple procedure has been effective in adults and children, even during serious attacks. "One of my first experiences as an apprentice herbalist with Susun Weed," Bennett told me, "was to smoke a mullein cigarette with her so that I could experience for myself the feeling of my bronchioles dilating in response to the soothing smoke. This is another traditional way of using mullein for asthma." Bennett's students report that drinking a strong mullein leaf infusion daily helps reduce the frequency and severity of asthma attacks. Some have successfully weaned themselves off all asthma medication, such as one runner who found herself able to complete her run without having to stop and use her inhaler. In addition, Bennett suggests the use of positive affirmations, such as "I deserve to breathe freely," as reminders that deep, comfortable, healthy breathing is each person's right. "Self-worth is often an issue," she explained. "Whatever a person can do to increase his or her self-esteem is a powerful treatment for asthma."

Bronchitis

Bronchitis is defined as an acute (intense and sudden) or chronic (longstanding) inflammation of the mucous lining of the bronchial tubes, the main airway to the lungs. Acute bronchitis often develops after an upper respiratory infection, such as a cold or the flu. The resulting cough is at first very dry but it becomes less painful and rasping as the lungs produce mucus, which lubricates the bronchi. In some cases, bronchitis may be followed by pneumonia. If a fever persists for more than a few days, complications are likely.

Statistics show that smokers are more likely to die from chronic bronchitis than from lung cancer, so for smokers, the best strategy is to quit.

Foods such as wheat (especially white flour), refined carbohydrates, sugar and dairy products often exacerbate chronic bronchitis. By experimenting with diet, eliminating processed foods, dairy products and wheat while increasing the consumption of raw foods, many have reduced or eliminated their bronchitis symptoms. Garlic is often recommended as a food supplement, along with vitamins, minerals and "green" foods such as wheat grass, barley grass, spirulina or chlorella.

Expectorant herbs are important for relief of the exhausting cough that comes with bronchitis, but the type of herb depends on the type of cough. For relief from a dry, hacking, irritating cough, use a relaxing expectorant such as **coltsfoot** or **lobelia**; for a wet cough, use a stimulating expectorant like **horehound** or **elecampane**.

The Austrian herbalist Maria Treben recommended breathing the steam from **coltsfoot** flowers and leaves to relieve bronchitis. Pour boiling water over fresh or dried coltsfoot, then drape a towel over your head and the bowl to retain the resulting steam. Treben also recommended taking coltsfoot syrup (see recipe on page 64) and bathing the feet in warm coltsfoot tea. See page 64 for information on the safety of coltsfoot.

In *An Elder's Herbal*, David Hoffmann recommended **osha** (*Ligusticum porterii*), a plant native to the American Southwest, as "an excellent specific in cases of tracheobronchitis." Osha root, which has a sharp and pungent taste, can be chewed for relief from coughs and sore throats. For all bronchitis symptoms, Hoffmann recommended a tea made of equal parts **mullein**, **coltsfoot**, **marshmallow** and **aniseed**; pour 1 cup boiling water over 2 teaspoons dried herbs and let stand, covered, for 10 minutes. Drink several cups daily.

For bronchitis accompanied by wet coughing, Hoffmann suggested 1 tablespoon of an expectorant tincture made of equal parts **elecampane**, **horehound**, **coltsfoot**, **goldenseal** and **echinacea**, taken 3 times daily.

Steam inhalations, described on page 48, are soothing in all stages of bronchitis. Add 1 teaspoon each of **chamomile blossoms**, **thyme** and **marjoram** to 2 cups boiling water, or add any of the following essential oils to a bowl of steaming water: **bergamot**, **eucalyptus**, **fir**, **lavender**, **peppermint**, **sage**, **sandalwood**, **tea tree oil**, **thyme** or **white pine**. **Peppermint oil** may be most effective in the early stages of bronchitis.

As the patient recovers from bronchitis, **coltsfoot**, **horehound** and **mullein** are especially useful, given as teas or tinctures several times daily.

Colds and Flu

We associate these viral diseases with winter or with a change of season, but you can catch a cold or the flu any time. What's the difference? Both cause respiratory distress, fever, coughing, headaches, sore throats, aching muscles and fatigue, but the flu (short for influenza) is usually more severe, faster developing and involves more of the body. Vomiting and diarrhea are common flu symptoms.

If you're serious about staying well, it makes sense to improve your diet, reduce the stress in your life and avoid the foods, drugs and pollutants that suppress immunity. These include sugars, junk foods and cigarettes, as well as chemicals, pesticides and air pollutants.

Left alone, most colds go away by themselves within a week, but with the help of certain herbs, your symptoms should disappear much faster.

Herbs That Can Help. Mention colds and flu to most herbalists and they will recommend **echinacea**. The purple cone flower, *Echinacea purpurea,* and its narrow leaved relative, *E. angustifolia,* have been shown to increase T-cell activity and related immune system activity. When taken in the early stages of illness, echinacea wards off viral infection and is most effective when taken frequently, in large doses, for brief periods.

Echinacea is often combined with **goldenseal** or **Oregon grape root,** both of which contain berberine, a strong antibiotic substance. Goldenseal enhances immune function by stimulating circulation to the spleen, toning the lymph system. Echinacea and goldenseal work well with **licorice root,** an herb that supports the immune system through its effect on the adrenal system. Tinctures containing these combinations are widely sold, or make your own for even better results.

I learned to appreciate echinacea and goldenseal when a wet blizzard soaked me to the skin. My teeth chattered so loudly my husband said they sounded like castanets, my bones felt frozen and I sneezed and coughed all over everything. Most unpleasant! Beginning in the afternoon, I took 1/4 teaspoon of a combined echinacea and goldenseal tincture every half hour plus a gram of vitamin C every hour until I fell asleep at midnight. The next morning, not only had every trace of illness disappeared but I felt better than I had in months. This strategy works best if used on the first day of cold symptoms.

Astragalus root is an increasingly popular Chinese herb used to flavor soups and rice dishes. Chinese research has shown it to increase activity of the immune system, and it's easy to add a piece to whatever you're cooking to boost winter immunity.

Feed Your Cold. Chicken soup has a long medicinal history, dating back to the 12th-century physician Moses Maimonides, who is said to have prescribed it for the Muslim sultan, Saladin. Chicken contains cistine, an amino acid that closely resembles acetylcysteine, which doctors prescribe for respiratory infections. In 1978, Marvin Sackner, M.D., a pulmonary specialist at Mount Sinai Medical School in Florida, conducted a now famous "chicken soup" study. Fifteen healthy men and women sipped hot chicken soup, hot water or cold water out of covered and uncovered containers, after which their mucus and air-flow rates were measured. Chicken soup and its vapors relieved congestion better than either the hot or cold water.

Irwin Ziment, M.D., a professor medicine at the University of California at Los Angeles and an authority on traditional remedies, prescribes spicy foods for colds, sinusitis, asthma, hay fever, emphysema and chronic bronchitis because peppers and other spices perform as well as many over-the-counter drugs, but without their adverse side effects. Dr. Ziment calls spicy chicken soup "the best cold remedy there is," especially when flavored with **garlic**, **onion**, **pepper**, **curry** or **chili peppers**. To prevent colds and flu, he prescribes a bowl of spicy chicken soup daily. Vegetarians can substitute miso, a Japanese fermented soy bean paste, for chicken in a similarly spicy broth.

Because viruses thrive in dry environments, liquids are an important treatment for colds and flu. The old adage, "milk makes mucus," has been verified by Australian scientists, who discovered that milk consumption encourages congestion and prevents the free flow of mucus, so milk is one liquid that should be avoided when treating a cold. However, yogurt has a proven track record as a preventer of hay fever, colds and flu. In a year-long controlled study of 120 young and elderly adults, six ounces of active-culture yogurt daily significantly reduced these illnesses. George Halpern, M.D., who conducted the study at the University of California at Davis, recommends eating yogurt daily for at least three months ahead of hay fever and cold seasons, as "it takes that long for sufficient gamma interferon to build up in your system." Acidophilus and other live culture supplements provide even more of the active bacteria that improve health and digestion. Check your health food store's refrigerator.

Andrew Weil, M.D., prefers natural remedies to pharmaceuticals and his favorite cold cure is **garlic**. "Eat several cloves of raw garlic at the first onset of symptoms," he recommends. "Cut it in chunks and swallow them whole like pills. If it gives you flatulence, eat less. I recommend one or two cloves of garlic to people who suffer from chronic or recurrent infections or low resistance to infection."

In The *Science and Art of Herbology*, her popular course on herbal medicine, Rosemary Gladstar describes how to make a syrup that helps prevent and cure bronchial inflammation, asthma, hay fever, colds and coughs. She wrote:

I learned how to make this formula many years ago and the story of how I learned it is one I'd like to share. Hari Das Baba was doing a series of small retreats in the Occidental Hills. We'd all gather round him to feel his wisdom, as he had not spoken words for years and years. Sometimes there would be questions and answers time and Hari Das would write his brilliant answers on the chalkboard. Believe me, I thought about all the questions I wanted to ask! I thought for days and finally my turn came. I asked my cosmic question in all earnestness: "What is the best recipe you know of for asthma and hay fever?" And this is the recipe he shared. It's excellent stuff. Make at least one or two quarts. You'll use it all!

To make the syrup, which treats colds and flu as effectively as it does hay fever and asthma, juice equal parts fresh **ginger root** and fresh **garlic cloves** in a juicer. Combine them in a saucepan and sweeten with just enough **honey** to thicken (1/4 to 1/2 cup honey per cup of juice). Warm the mixture slightly to mix in the honey; do not heat. Remove from the stove and add enough **cayenne pepper** to make it taste hot, sweet, spicy and pungent at the same time. Pour the mixture into a glass jar and wrap it in a blanket or large towel and cover it with a paper bag. Find an appropriate place in or near your garden, dig a hole and bury the jar for 17 days. At the end of this time, it is ready to use. Suggested dosage: 1 teaspoon three times daily, as needed.

When I first made the garlic-ginger syrup, I seasoned it with tobasco sauce and left it buried in the ground for four months, a variation on the guru's recipe. Something definitely happened to change the ingredients; fermentation and the passage of time produced a stunning blend of flavors. In fact, my husband used it to season his stir-fried rice. When a friend had a cold that wouldn't go away, complete with a hacking cough that left his throat raw, we gave him an 8-ounce bottle. Taking a swig every half hour, he finished the bottle in one night. By morning, his cold had disappeared without a trace. Even his sore throat felt fine. Warning: the garlic odor is overwhelming, but when you really want to feel better, that doesn't matter.

If you don't have four months or even 17 days to spare, you can get relief from the same ingredients in other ways. The fresh juices of **garlic** and **ginger** combined with **honey** and **cayenne** will help chase away just about any viral infection, and so will garlic in foods, ginger in tea and cayenne pepper capsules. Ginger and cayenne are warming, stimulant herbs. They work well in combination with other herbs and can be added to any treatment involving capsules, tinctures and/or teas.

For additional cough relief suggestions, see pages 43–44.

To treat the sinus congestion that accompanies colds and flu, see the instructions for nasal rinsing, facial steam treatments and ginger fomentations on pages 47, 48 and 58.

To relieve a sore throat, see page 49.

To treat chest congestion, see the directions for making a mustard plaster and mustard bath on page 77. You can also combine congestion-clearing essential oils with a carrier oil such as olive or almond oil to make a soothing chest balm. **Peppermint, eucalyptus, tea tree, wintergreen, cinnamon** and **clove oils** all work well for this purpose. Be sure to dilute these essential oils in a carrier oil before applying them to the skin, for full strength oils can cause irritation or blisters.

Coughs

Coughing is a reflex response to anything that interferes with the passage of air to the lungs. In most cases, the cause is mucus secreted by membranes lining the respiratory tract.

The breathless cough of an asthma attack can be treated with **mullein**, including the smoke of a burning mullein leaf (see page 36). When anxiety contributes to asthma, relaxing nervines such as **oatstraw, chamomile** and **lobelia** help prevent spasms and coughing.

As noted in the section describing bronchitis, dry, hacking, irritating coughs respond well to relaxing expectorants like **lobelia** and **coltsfoot**, while wet coughs need more stimulating expectorants such as **horehound** and **elecampane**.

Any cough can be soothed by chewing on **osha root** (see page 79) or, especially recommended for smokers, **calamus root** (page 62).

When an illness such as a cold or the flu causes coughing, the use of cough-suppressing herbs interferes with the body's cleansing mechanisms, for coughing helps the body rid itself of waste products. In that case, expectorant herbs such as **horehound** and **coltsfoot** are effective, for they make coughing more productive. Infection-fighting herbs such as **echinacea** and the culinary herbs **sage** and **thyme** are also helpful, for they help remove the cause of the illness.

Whenever coughing produces blood or does not respond to treatment and lasts more than a week, it should be checked by a medical professional.

Herbalist Gail Ulrich uses the following cough syrup for colds, flu and other respiratory problems.

First, blend equal parts **wild cherry bark, licorice root** and **burdock root**, then add a smaller amount (1/4 to 1/2 part) **osha root**. In a quart jar place 2 tablespoons of this herbal blend, cover with boiling water, close the jar and let the tea steep for at least 4 hours or overnight.

Next, blend equal parts of **dried mullein leaf**, **sage**, **coltsfoot** and **comfrey leaf**, then add a small amount (1/4 part) **peppermint** and, for adults, an equal amount of **horehound**. Place 2 tablespoons of this tea in a quart Mason jar, add boiling water, close the lid and let the tea stand for 2 hours.

Strain and combine these two teas in a large sauce pan and simmer, uncovered, until the tea is reduced to 1/2 or (for a stronger syrup) 1/4 of its volume. For every cup of tea add 3 to 4 tablespoons honey or a combination of 2 tablespoons honey and 2 tablespoons black cherry concentrate. Add a splash of brandy as a preservative and use as needed to soothe a sore throat.

To make old-fashioned horehound candy cough drops, see the recipe on page 69. See page 64 for a coltsfoot cough syrup recipe, page 76 for marshmallow root cough syrup and page 50 for a cayenne pepper taffy that soothes sore throats.

Croup

An affliction of young children, usually between six months and two years of age, croup is an inflammation and obstruction of the larynx that often follows a viral infection of the respiratory tract. A painful, honking cough, harsh breathing, rising pulse rate, restlessness and irritability are common but alarming symptoms. So is cyanosis, a bluish tint in the skin caused by oxygen deprivation.

In orthodox medicine, croup is treated with humidification and mild sedatives. The herbal therapy is similar. A steam vaporizer containing a few drops of **eucalyptus**, **tea tree**, **sage** or **thyme** essential oil helps bring relief, especially if left on overnight. Warm lemonade, fresh juices diluted with water and **chamomile** tea are all recommended. **Lobelia** is a powerful muscle relaxer that can be added in tea or tincture form to any liquid the child will take. In fact, any of the relaxing nervines will help, including **chamomile, oatstraw** and **valerian**. Massaging the chest with an aromatic balm is also recommended.

Earaches

Aching ears aren't really a respiratory condition, but earaches often accompany colds, hay fever or allergy attacks and sinus infections. They are especially common in small children, and children treated with antibiotics usually suffer recurring infections.

If treated at the onset of symptoms such as rubbing the ears, irritability, fussiness or complaints of ear pain, infections can be avoided. Buy or make an ear oil using **olive oil, garlic** and/or **mullein flowers** (see page 58). Warm the oil to a comfortable temperature and drop a few drops down each ear 6 to 10 times daily. Warm oil is the most widely recommended therapy for ear pain.

Because diet is so often implicated in ear infections, Rosemary Gladstar recommends that all congestion-causing foods be avoided (her list includes eggs, dairy, wheat and sugar in all forms) by infected children and their nursing mothers.

Any relaxing tea, such as **chamomile** or **oatstraw**, will be helpful, as are teas containing infection-fighting herbs such as **echinacea** and **goldenseal**.

Emphysema

Now known officially as chronic obstructive pulmonary disease or COPD, emphysema often accompanies chronic bronchitis. It is caused by a lack of elasticity in the lungs, usually due to constant coughing. When the lungs cannot expand and contract with ease, it is difficult breathe. Emphysema often brings a distinctive deep wheezing that interrupts conversation and physical movement. It is so debilitating that it ranks third among the diseases for which Social Security gives disability benefits. Patients often have a history of heavy smoking or live in areas of high air pollution.

The herbal treatments for emphysema are similar to those for asthma, with an added emphasis on nutritional support for the immune system. See the suggestions for asthma therapy. Some physicians prescribe a low-carbohydrate diet because sweets, simple carbohydrates and sugar tend to worsen emphysema symptoms. In 1992 British researchers published a double-blind, randomized crossover study to test the effects of fats and carbohydrates on emphysema. They found that small dietary changes in the balance of carbohydrates to fats affected exercise tolerance and breathlessness significantly. The more carbohydrates the patients consumed, the worse their symptoms.

Vitamins C and E, magnesium and bioflavonids are important supplements for those with emphysema and so are omega-3 fish oils. In 1994, the *New England Journal of Medicine* reported on a study of nearly 9,000 smokers and former smokers that showed the more fish they ate, the less chance they had of developing emphysema.

In the 1950s, Robert Atkins, M.D., served as a medical resident in the Columbia Chest Division of Bellevue Hospital in New York City. This division was dedicated to the treatment of emphysema and was run by two Nobel Prize winners. As Dr. Atkins explained in the November 1995 issue of his *Health Revelations* newsletter, oxygen had always been known to benefit people who had emphysema or COPD, but doctors administered it intermittently, fearing that a supplemental supply would signal the brain that it need not breathe so often. However, several studies have shown that patients do well when oxygen is administered continuously, especially at night. Two trials in the 1980s showed a 50 percent improvement in the rate of death when people with COPD received continuous oxygen therapy.

Smoking is a major cause of emphysema. The relaxing expectorant herbs **lobelia** and **coltsfoot** can be helpful in treating emphysema, as can **bloodroot** and **elecampane**. For example, a tea made of equal parts coltsfoot, lobelia and the soothing demulcent herbs **mullein** and **Irish moss** may help reduce coughing and shortness of breath. Add an equal amount of **licorice root** if high blood pressure and fluid retention are not a problem. Use 1 to 2 teaspoons tea per cup of boiling water; brew 4 cups at a time in a quart jar for convenience, reheat as desired and sip throughout the day.

See *Coughs* on page 43 for additional suggestions.

Laryngitis

An inflammation of the larynx or vocal cords, laryngitis causes hoarseness and, in serious cases, loss of voice. The best treatments for laryngitis are silence (don't even try to talk) and the passage of time. Steam treatments like those used for sinusitis are recommended. In addition, gargle with **sage tea** or **salt water**. The relaxing nervines, especially **lobelia**, **oatstraw** and **chamomile**, soothe frazzled nerves as well as inflamed tissue.

For pain relief, see the *Sore Throat* suggestions on pages 49–50.

Sinus Congestion

A symptom of hay fever allergies and colds or flu, sinus congestion makes breathing difficult. Chronic sinusitis sometimes follows these illnesses, causing a dull ache around the eyes and face.

To relieve sinus congestion, rinse the nasal passages with a solution of warm water and unrefined sea salt. Swimming in the ocean is one way to relieve congestion; another is to create the same effect while standing over the bathroom sink. Hand-held ceramic containers with long spouts have become popular for this purpose; see the Neti Pot in the appendix. Similar designs are available in some health food stores and catalogs. If you can't find a Neti Pot, ask your pharmacist for a nasal douche apparatus or simply hold salt water in your hand and sniff it up one nostril while you hold the other closed. The more salt water that irrigates sinus passages, the greater the relief. Use enough so that the water drains out through your mouth, washing away debris as it does.

To disinfect as you rinse, add a few drops of **grapefruit seed** or **citrus seed extract** to the salt solution. Grapefruit seed extract kills bacteria, viruses, yeasts, molds, parasites, fungi and other pathogens on contact. Another therapy recommended by naturopaths is to rinse the nasal passages with **goldenseal tea**. Be sure the tea is warm, not hot, and add a pinch of salt to make the rinsing more comfortable and effective. Alternatively, add a pinch of salt to warm **sage** or **thyme tea**.

Facial steam baths help clear sinus passages and allow free breathing. This therapy can be as simple as holding your head over a steaming bowl of chicken soup when you have a cold. If you have a facial sauna, sold in beauty supply shops and some pharmacies, plug it in and inhale. For an aromatherapy treatment, pour boiling water into a bowl to which you have added a few drops of congestion-relieving essential oils, such as **eucalyptus**, **sage**, **rosemary**, **ginger** or **tea tree oil**, or use **chamomile tea**. Make a tent of a large towel to cover your head and the bowl, then breathe the medicated steam for several minutes. Keep your head well above the bowl to prevent scalding, and come out for air as necessary.

See the instructions for making a sinus-clearing ginger fomentation on page 58.

The herbs **Ma huang** and **goldenseal** are specifics for sinus problems. Astringent herbs such as **goldenrod**, **eyebright** and **elderflowers** contain tannins that help dry up excess mucus. **Echinacea** and **garlic** fight upper respiratory infections. And don't forget diet. A major cause of chronic sinusitis is food sensitivities. In addition to using herbs that help relieve symptoms, a new diet may eliminate the condition altogether.

Sore Throat

The pain of a sore throat makes any illness worse. One traditional treatment is to gargle with salt water or a strong herbal tea several times a day, spitting the gargle solution out without swallowing. Add a teaspoon of salt to a cup of water or warm tea for this purpose. If you can sing and gargle at the same time, the soothing liquid will contact more throat surface.

Licorice root tea soothes throat soreness and reduces pain. Simmer 1 tablespoon licorice root in 3 cups water, covered, for 10-15 minutes. Drink one cup three times daily unless you have high blood pressure or edema (fluid retention). Gargling with licorice root tea does not cause side effects.

Hot **sage tea** is a popular European remedy for sore throats. Steep 1 or 2 teaspoons **dried sage** leaves or 1 to 2 tablespoons fresh sage in 1 cup boiling water, covered, for 10 minutes. Sip slowly or add salt and gargle.

Horseradish mixed with **honey**, water and **ground cloves** is an old Russian remedy for sore throat. Mix 1 tablespoon grated fresh horseradish, 1 teaspoon honey and 1 teaspoon ground cloves in a glass of warm water until blended. Stir often and sip slowly or use as a gargle.

Capsaicin, the active ingredient in cayenne peppers, is so effective at preventing pain that it is used to treat the mouth sores of people taking chemotherapy or radiation treatments for cancers of the head and neck. Researchers at Yale University developed a chile pepper taffy for patients with mouth lesions resulting from orthodox cancer treatments and it works as well for throat pain brought on by colds or flu. The

following recipe was published in the May 1996 issue of
Chile Pepper magazine.

In a 2-quart saucepan, combine 1 cup sugar, 1/4 cup light
corn syrup, 2/3 cup water, 1 tablespoon cornstarch, 2 tablespoons butter and 1 teaspoon salt. Cook over medium heat
to the hard ball stage (265 degrees Fahrenheit on a candy
thermometer, or until a small amount dropped into very cold
water forms a hard ball). Remove from heat, stir in 2 teaspoons vanilla and 1/2 teaspoon powdered cayenne pepper and
pour into a buttered pan. When it's cool enough to handle
(this part is easier with two people), lightly butter your hands
and pull the taffy until it is satiny, light in color and stiff.
Pull it into long strips 1/2-inch wide and cut the strips into 1-
inch pieces. Wrap pieces individually in waxed paper and store
them in an airtight container. This recipe makes about a pound
of taffy.

Of course, you can adapt the recipe, substituting 2/3 cup
strong herbal tea for the water, using any throat-friendly
herb.

HERBS FOR THE PULMONARY SYSTEM

There are many ways to classify herbs, which is why the vocabulary of herbalists is so rich with descriptive terms like expectorant, demulcent, stimulant and nervine. Here are the categories that deal with respiratory conditions.

Anticatarrhal herbs heal the chronic inflammation of respiratory mucous membranes. They prevent the buildup of excess mucus. Examples include cayenne pepper, sage, goldenseal, mullein, ginger, echinacea and garlic.

Antispasmodic herbs relax cramping muscles. Pulmonary antispasmodics have a special affinity for the respiratory system and are most helpful in treating asthma. Lobelia and wild cherry bark are examples.

Demulcent herbs are by definition soothing. They coat irritated, inflamed tissue with mucilage and reduce coughing by relaxing bronchial tension. Examples include Iceland moss, lungwort, plantain and pleurisy root.

Expectorant herbs stimulate the removal of mucus from the lungs, and they often have a tonic effect on the whole respiratory system. Some expectorants work by irritating the bronchioles, speeding the ejection of mucoid material; others work by relaxing or soothing bronchial passages, reducing spasms and relieving dry, irritating coughs. Stimulating expectorants include horehound and elecampane; relaxing expectorants include coltsfoot, lobelia and mullein.

Nervines are relaxing herbs that strengthen and nourish the nervous system. They are useful in treating asthma and hay fever, and they help anyone suffering from a respiratory problem that prevents rest and sleep. Hyssop, motherwort and lobelia are respiratory nervines.

Tonic herbs nurture the system and help the body correct whatever is out of balance. Pulmonary tonics offer special benefits to the lungs and respiratory system; examples include elecampane and mullein.

A **specific** for a particular condition is an herb known for its beneficial effects, such as mullein or lobelia for asthma or Ma huang (ephedra) for hay fever. Specifics can be used alone or combined with other herbs, in which case they act as the blend's active ingredient.

A **catalyst** or **activator** herb is often used in herbal blends to stimulate increased circulation and digestion, speeding the action of the herbs it accompanies. Some stimulant herbs are used alone in the treatment of respiratory complaints, such as Ma huang, but most make up a small portion of an herbal recipe. Lobelia and ginger are examples of catalyst herbs added in small doses to many teas and tinctures. Cayenne pepper helps the respiratory system, but its hot taste makes therapeutic doses difficult to take by mouth. For this reason, some herbalists recommend taking a cayenne pepper capsule while drinking a tea that you hope will bring fast relief. Another powerful catalyst herb is horseradish, which has cleared plenty of sinuses, as has another warming herb, mustard.

The most widely used stimulant herb in America is caffeine, and while it is not usually recommended by herbalists, caffeine does increase circulation and speed the distribution of chemicals through the body. Cayenne pepper, ginger and lobelia are less dramatic in action and can be used in any combination of herbs at any time of the day or night.

Herbal Preparations. There are many ways to take herbs: in teas, capsules, tablets, syrups, lozenges and tinctures, not to mention all their external applications, like compresses, poultices, washes and steam inhalations.

For best results, use herbs that were grown organically or wildcrafted, then dried at low temperature to maintain their flavor, color, essential oils and other properties. See the appendix for a list of herbal tea companies that specialize in high quality medicinal herbs.

If you are new to herbal medicine, remember that the recipes given here and in herbal reference books are flexible and forgiving. If you can't obtain an ingredient, find an appropriate substitute. Quantities are flexible, too. As you gain experience, you will be able to develop your own recipes. As you do so, be sure to refer to two or three different herbal references for information about each plant so that you have a clear understanding of its benefits, potential side effects and special requirements.

Teas. To brew a tea of fresh or dried leaves or blossoms, use 1 to 2 teaspoons dry herb or 1 to 2 tablespoons fresh herb per cup of water. Bring the water to a boil, pour it over the herbs, cover the teapot or container with a lid and let it stand undisturbed for 10 minutes. This type of tea is called an *infusion*. Some plants are so delicate that herbalists recommend using cold instead of hot water, a brewing process that requires several hours.

To make a *cold-water infusion,* shred or chop the plant material before placing it in a small but roomy muslin bag or folded cotton handkerchief. Tie the fabric with string so that the herbs don't escape, but leave enough space inside for water to circulate. Dampen the herbs with cold water as you fill a quart jar, and when you close the jar, suspend the bag near the top. Leave the jar undisturbed overnight. As plant material is extracted by the water, solids fall to the bottom of the jar, creating a rising current that moves through the herbs. This is the most effective type of cold infusion you can make. Alternatively, simply mix plant material with cold water in any container and let it stand overnight. In the morning, strain the tea and heat it slightly, just enough to warm it, before serving.

To brew a *decoction* (boiled tea) from roots, bark or other hard, woody material, use the quantities given above and place the herbs and cold water in a stainless steel pan, cover and heat to the boiling point. Lower the heat, simmer the tea for 10 to 15 minutes, then remove from heat and let stand another 5 minutes before straining and serving.

Medicinal herbs can be sweetened with honey to improve their taste, or you can add flavors such as black cherry concentrate or fresh ginger or a pinch of stevia, the sweet herb widely used as a sugar substitute. Most herbalists recommend taking medicinal teas straight, with no added flavors or sweeteners. Add a pinch of unrefined, unprocessed sea salt to herbal teas when treating sinus or chest congestion or a sore throat.

Tinctures. To make a tincture, which is a concentrated alcohol extract, fill a glass jar 1/3 to 1/2 full with fresh or dried herbs that you have cut or shredded into small pieces. Cover the herbs with 80-proof or higher proof vodka, rum, brandy or grain alcohol, with a few inches of alcohol above the plant matter. Cover tightly and place in a warm location. Check the jar every day or two, shaking it as you do so. As dried herbs absorb the liquid, add more alcohol. (Some recipes call for 1 part plant matter to 4 parts alcohol, but using less alcohol or more plant material results in a more concentrated, medicinal tincture.) Let the tincture stand for three or four weeks before filtering. Some herbalists recommend straining and bottling tinctures at the full moon. There is no specific deadline; a tincture left for two months will be more potent than one left for two weeks. Strain the tincture through cheesecloth or muslin, pressing out as much liquid as possible before discarding the spent plant material. Alcohol tinctures have an indefinite shelf life. Stored in amber glass jars away from heat and light, they last for decades.

For an even more concentrated tincture, pour your filtered tincture into a jar containing new plant material and repeat the process. Small quantities of this "double-strength" tincture will have a powerful medicinal effect.

There is much confusion about tincture dosage, a misunderstanding that herbalist Rosemary Gladstar attributes to the caution of small companies marketing tinctures in the 1960s. "The only similar products were homeopathic preparations," she explains, "and their doses are measured in drops. Herbal tinctures are entirely different, and they should be taken by the half-teaspoon, teaspoon or tablespoon, not by the drop." Anyone buying, making or taking herbal tinctures should know that disappointing results may not be caused by a tincture's herbal ingredients but rather by doses that are entirely too small. A few herbs should be taken in small doses, but most of the tinctures mentioned here are safe and effective in larger doses. Tinctures can be taken straight or diluted in tea, water or fruit juice.

If you prefer not to use alcohol in tincture making, vegetable glycerine can be substituted, or you can mix glycerine with alcohol. Glycerine does not dissolve all of the medicinal constituents that alcohol extracts, but it is widely used in tinctures, especially for children. Glycerine adds a sweet taste and syrupy texture to tinctures. Cider vinegar can be used to make alcohol-free tinctures, though their shelf life is shorter than glycerine or alcohol tinctures and vinegar does not dissolve as many substances within the herbs.

Capsules. Herbal capsules are widely sold and, if you need a special blend of herbs into capsules, some of the mail order herb companies blend and encapsulate custom orders for a nominal fee. Or you can put your own herbs in capsules. For best results, leave dried herbs whole or in large pieces until needed, to preserve their essential oils and medicinal properties. Herbs should be stored away from heat and light in well-sealed glass containers for maximum shelf life. When ready to use, grind them in a blender or spice grinder until they are powdered. To reduce exposure to herb dust, which can irritate nasal passages, wear a pollen mask. Two-part gelatin capsules, including vegetable gelatin capsules for vegetarians, are widely sold in health food stores and herb catalogs in sizes ranging from 0 (largest) to 00 and 000 (smallest). Many herbal companies sell mechanical capping devices that hold several capsules in place for faster and easier filling.

Poultices and Plasters. A *poultice* is a wet herbal pack applied directly to an inflamed, irritated, swollen, infected or injured part of the body. While poultices are often made of fresh mashed herbs, they can also be made of the residue left after brewing tea. Poultices are usually applied cool rather than hot. Some herbalists recommend spreading a thin layer of olive oil or castor oil before applying the plant material. Use whatever will hold the poultice in place for several hours: bandages, plastic wrap, cheesecloth, muslin, etc. An elastic elbow brace or knee bandage can hold a poultice in place on arms and lower legs. A layer of plastic over the poultice helps prevent fabric stains.

A *plaster* is a dry poultice made by spreading dry powdered herbs, or a thick paste made by adding a small amount of water over cotton or muslin fabric. Additional fabric is spread over the skin to protect it, as most of the herbs used for plasters can be irritating to the skin, such as mustard or cayenne. The plaster is held in place for several minutes, then lifted so the skin can be checked, and replaced if the skin isn't irritated. Plasters increase circulation and help clear congestion.

Compresses and Fomentations.

A *compress* is an application of cold herbal tea on a saturated towel, diaper or thick cloth. Use medicinal strength infusions or decoctions for this purpose. To treat a fever, chill a strong peppermint tea, then soak the cloth and wring it just until it stops dripping. The compress should be wet enough to stay cold for several minutes. When it warms to body temperature, soak it again, adding ice as needed to keep the tea cold. Repeat until the treatment has lasted 15 to 20 minutes. Dry the skin gently.

Chamomile tea bags are an example of cold compresses. For sore or swollen eyes, brew strong chamomile tea using two or more teabags and just enough boiling water to cover them. Let stand, covered, until cool; add ice or store in the freezer or refrigerator until cold. Then lie down, relax and place a saturated tea bag over each eye. Alternatively, brew strong chamomile tea, strain it through cheesecloth or a paper coffee filter, chill it, then saturate cotton makeup-removal pads, cotton balls, a washcloth, cheesecloth or other fabric and apply the compress. Repeat as desired to relieve the itchy swelling of eyes during hay fever, colds or allergies.

A *fomentation* is a hot compress. Fomentations increase circulation and help clear respiratory congestion. Wearing rubber gloves, saturate a thick cloth with strong, hot, strained tea; wring it gently, then unfold it to let it cool slightly. You don't want it to burn or scald, but for best results it must be as hot as possible. Test the temperature against your inner arm. When it's hot but not too hot, apply it to the desired area and cover with a thick folded towel to retain heat.

peat after 5 or 10 minutes. For best results, reapply for 15 to 30 minutes. Obviously, this and any other treatment should be discontinued if the person becomes uncomfortable or if the skin becomes irritated.

A strong decoction of fresh grated ginger can be applied to the sinus area to clear congestion. For extra benefit, try adding a pinch of powdered mustard or a few drops of eucalyptus, wintergreen or tea tree oil.

Oil Infusions To make an oil infusion, such as an oil for treating ear infections or an aromatic rub to relieve chest congestion, you can use the stove, an oven or the sun (solar infusion).

Fresh chopped garlic and fresh or dried mullein blossoms are traditional ingredients in ear oils. Use either or any combination of both. For an aromatic chest rub oil, use any combination of fresh or dried wintergreen, eucalyptus, peppermint, whole cayenne pepper pods, whole mustard seed, cinnamon sticks, whole cloves or cracked whole nutmegs.

Cover the plant material with olive oil and heat it gently in the top of a double boiler above simmering water or in a closed glass jar set on a rack in a pan of simmering water for one to two hours or longer. If using dry herbs, additional oil may be needed as the plant matter absorbs it. Use enough oil to cover the herbs well but not so much that your result is weak and ineffective. Start with 2 cups oil to 1 cup dried herbs and adjust the proportions as desired. Fresh herbs will absorb less liquid, so simply cover them with oil.

To make a *solar infusion,* which is my favorite method, let fresh plant material wilt slightly to reduce water content, use a clean jar, loosely pack the jar with fresh herbs (fill the jar half full if using dried herbs), then fill it to the top with oil, clean the top of the jar well so that no oil or plant material interferes with a tight seal when you put the lid on and leave the jar outside in the sun for several weeks or months.

When ready to use, strain through cheesecloth and add a few drops of tea tree oil or grapefruit seed extract as a disinfecting preservative. If you're making an aromatic chest rub, add a few drops of decongesting eucalyptus oil as well. Store in amber glass bottles (use an eye dropper bottle for ear oil) away from heat and light. Label with ingredients and date of preparation. Stored correctly, oils can last for years, though most herbalists prefer to make them annually for maximum freshness. Note that these oils are for external use only. Discard any oil that becomes rancid.

Dosages. Most of the herbs recommended for respiratory conditions are safe to take in teas, tinctures, syrups, capsules, tablets or lozenges several times daily for several days or weeks at a time. Note the safety issues raised about bloodroot, coltsfoot, comfrey, lobelia and calamus root and the potential side effects of Ma huang and licorice root, all of which are discussed in the following section.

The tincture doses that appear on the labels of dropper bottles sold in health food stores, usually measured in drops, are insufficient for most acute conditions in adult humans. Also, many commercially prepared tinctures are weaker and less concentrated than those you can make at home, either because the proportion of alcohol to herbs is higher, creating a more dilute solution; because the tinctures are made quickly, allowing insufficient time for complete extraction; or because the quality of the raw materials is inferior.

Because concentration and quality vary among tinctures, just as the people who take them vary in size, weight and physical condition, it is impossible to specify a single dosage for best results. If you don't notice improvement after taking a tincture as directed, you probably need more. As noted earlier, herbalists such as Rosemary Gladstar recommend teaspoon-sized doses of tinctures, not 7 to 15 drops at a time as many labels suggest. Of course, a one-ounce bottle won't last long if you take it a teaspoon at a time, which is why it makes sense to make your own.

In general, if you purchase a tincture that is clear in color and has no distinctive herbal taste or smell, it is less likely to be effective than one made of the same herb that has a strong taste, smell and color.

If you purchase capsules, try to buy them from a retailer whose stock rotates quickly or who powders herbs for capsules as needed. Powdered herbs lose their potency when exposed to heat, light or humidity.

As you become familiar with herbs, experiment with small doses of single herbs in tea, tinctures or capsules before taking therapeutic doses—several cups of medicinal strength tea, for example, a dozen capsules a day or a teaspoon of tincture three times daily. If you are allergic to an herb or have any adverse reaction to it, substitute something else. Adverse reactions to the herbs recommended here are unusual, but they can and do happen.

THE HERBAL PHARMACY

BLOODROOT *(Sanguinaria canadensis)*. Few Americans recognize its name, but millions start their day with it, for Sanguinaria extract is the active ingredient in Viadent toothpaste and mouthwash. A native American plant, bloodroot is a powerful expectorant that relaxes bronchial muscles. Because it helps clear chronic congestion of the lungs, it is a specific for bronchitis and emphysema; in addition, it supports the treatment of laryngitis, asthma and croup. Bloodroot is an ingredient in some herbal blends designed to treat these illnesses, and the dried rhizome can be purchased separately as a tea or tincture.

Bloodroot's potential toxicity is its only drawback. Although no cases of poisoning have been reported, even small doses have resulted in headaches, nausea and vomiting. James Duke, Ph.D., the widely respected and recently retired botanical expert at the U.S. Department of Agriculture, nibbled a small piece and experienced tunnel vision. David Hoffmann recommends a maximum of 3 cups of tea daily, made as a decoction from 1 teaspoon dried rhizome, or no more than 1/4 teaspoon tincture 3 times a day. As with any herb, discontinue use if you experience discomfort. Consult an herbalist or healthcare professional before giving bloodroot preparations to children.

Calamus Root or Sweet Flag (Acorus calamus).

An aromatic bitter, demulcent and antispasmodic, sweet flag or calamus root is widely used in Europe for indigestion, but it is also an important herb for those who want to quit smoking. Chewing the dried root stimulates saliva and has a calming effect on the respiratory tract. In her encyclopedic *Modern Herbal,* Mrs. M. Grieves wrote, "The rhizome is largely used in native Oriental medicines for dyspepsia and bronchitis and chewed as a cough lozenge." Calamus root is recommended for smokers because it stimulates salivation while having a tonic effect on the mucous membrane lining of the mouth and throat.

Calamus root was featured on the FDA's List of Unsafe Herbs, which was discontinued years ago because of its inaccuracies, and it is still listed in the U.S. Code of Federal Regulations as prohibited from direct addition to or use in human food. The controversy over calamus root stems from its asarone, a compound found to be carcinogenic in laboratory rats when taken in large quantities. Dr. Rudolf Weiss, the German authority on herbal medicine, wrote that calamus root has been popular from antiquity and is still widely used in Europe today without any reports of it causing cancer or any other problems. In *The New Age Herbalist,* Richard Mabey wrote that rhizomes from Europe have low concentrations of asarone compared with those from India, and no cases of malignancy have been reported in mill and mine workers who chew the rhizome daily. A conservative approach is to verify the source of calamus root and use this highly effective herb for short periods when needed.

The volatile oils in calamus root are so fragile that Maria Treben recommended brewing calamus tea with cold water. Those same volatile oils, when released by steam, can be a pleasant, soothing, aromatic therapy for upper respiratory congestion. Pour boiling water over calamus root and inhale its sweet, spicy vapors. Because few health food stores carry calamus root, it may have to be ordered from an herb company. The rhizome has many aromatherapy uses and can be used as a sachet to scent sheets, pillowcases and clothing. It is also a popular ingredient in potpourris.

Cayenne Pepper *(Capsicum annuum).* The familiar hot chile pepper, cayenne has a host of medicinal uses. Although usually considered a circulatory and digestive stimulant, cayenne has respiratory benefits as well. In addition to having a tonic and warming effect on the entire body, cayenne has expectorant properties and helps relieve winter colds, congestion and inflammation. Because it combines well with other herbs, cayenne makes an effective catalyst that enhances its companions' medicinal properties. The most comfortable way to take cayenne pepper is in capsules. For best results, take cayenne capsules with plenty of food and water. The first few times you do so, you may experience a burning sensation in the chest or stomach. To avoid this, take peppermint tea at the same time, eat an apple, drink apple juice or simply take cayenne pepper more often. The cayenne capsules sold in health food stores are of low to medium heat strength, so they are safe for most people to take several times daily. Adventurous herbalists experiment with their own blends of Scotch bonnets, Thai chiles, African birdseye and other really hot peppers in capsules. For an excellent and entertaining book about the adventures of one man who credits cayenne pepper with saving his life, read *Left for Dead* by Dick Quinn.

Chamomile *(Matricaria chamomilla or M. recutita).* Chamomile is more often prescribed for digestive disorders, insomnia and frazzled nerves than for respiratory problems, but this soothing, fragrant tea is helpful whenever stress, tension or nervousness adds to the symptoms of asthma and other breathing problems. Steam releases chamomile's essential oils to the mucous membranes of the lungs and sinuses, and chamomile tea with a pinch of sea salt makes an effective decongestant rinse for nasal passages. See instructions for using chamomile tea as a cold compress on page 57.

Coltsfoot (Tussilago farfara). This important herb for the respiratory system is considered a specific for chronic or acute bronchitis, irritating coughs, whooping cough, asthma, emphysema, laryngitis, bronchial asthma and even tuberculosis. Combining a soothing expectorant effect with antispasmodic action, coltsfoot reduces inflammation and promotes free breathing. According to Mrs. Grieves, smoking the dried leaves of coltsfoot has been recommended for relief from coughs since ancient times. Jethro Kloss, another legendary herbalist, recommended snuffing powdered leaves up the nostrils for nasal obstructions and headaches. Rudolf Weiss prescribed hot coltsfoot tea for emphysema and morning cough, recommending a cup before rising. Maria Treben wrote that inhaling steam from the flowers and leaves soothes bronchitis and relieves shortness of breath.

In 1987, a Swiss infant born with a severely damaged liver died. Every day of her pregnancy, the mother drank an expectorant tea containing coltsfoot. The tea contained *senecionine,* a pyrrolizidine alkaloid, but its source was uncertain; it may not have been coltsfoot. As a precaution, the German government placed a one-year moratorium on the sale of coltsfoot. No other cases of potential coltsfoot toxicity were discovered and the ban was repealed.

Syrups for respiratory conditions are easy to make and use. For example, to make an effective cough syrup, combine 2 tablespoons each of dried coltsfoot, echinacea, wild cherry bark, slippery elm bark, sage, horehound and ginger in 2 cups water. Simmer the herbs for about an hour over low to medium heat, uncovered, until half the water has evaporated. Strain the tea through cheesecloth and add an equal amount of raw honey or brown rice syrup.

It's more exotic, but I'm partial to the following recipe

for coltsfoot leaf syrup from Maria Treben's book *Health through God's Pharmacy*. Treben recommended this syrup for all lung disorders, coughs and bronchitis. In a large ceramic pot or glass jar, alternate layers of fresh coltsfoot leaves and raw sugar, let it settle and keep adding more until the pot is full. Wrap the pot in newspaper or fabric, then dig a hole in the garden and bury it. After eight weeks, dig it up and strain the syrup into a large pan and bring it just to a boil. Pour it into small jars. "This syrup is our best protection against winter and influenza," wrote Treben. "Take it in teaspoonful doses."

Coltsfoot is the first herb to bloom in the Northeast and I'm always cheered by its yellow blossoms rising through the snow in early spring. Adapting Treben's recipe, I have made wonderful coltsfoot syrups using raw sugar or a blend of raw sugar and raw honey layered with freshly picked coltsfoot leaves in a large glass jar which I leave outdoors in the sun all summer. From time to time I turn the tightly sealed jar upside down so its liquid contents can circulate. Instead of boiling the syrup, I simply strain it into clean glass jars and store them in a cool, dark place. This year I'm experimenting with coltsfoot-ginger syrup using sliced fresh ginger root, another soothing remedy for sore throats and chronic coughs.

Comfrey (Symphytum officinale). Comfrey is a powerful respiratory healer, thanks to its demulcent, anti-inflammatory and expectorant properties. In addition, comfrey contains allantoin, a cell-growth stimulator that makes it an effective treatment for cuts and wounds. It even speeds the healing of broken bones.

Comfrey is a specific in the treatment of bronchitis and irritable, painful coughs, for it soothes inflamed tissue, reduces irritation and relieves congestion.

But comfrey is a controversial herb and many health food stores no longer carry it. Comfrey contains a class of compounds that, when isolated and fed to laboratory rats in large doses, can cause liver damage. For hundreds of years, comfrey has been among the most widely used medicinal herbs in Europe and the United States with no adverse side effects ever reported. However, in 1984 a woman who had been taking comfrey-pepsin tablets developed liver toxicity and soon warnings of every description appeared in the media. Since then, three additional cases of liver disease have been found in people who took comfrey. Because of the laboratory rat test results and because the FDA has published warnings about the herb based on these four cases, some herbalists no longer recommend comfrey. However, since none of the four human cases of liver disease were proved to be caused by comfrey and because thousands of tons of the herb have been consumed by hundreds of thousands of people with only good results reported, others continue to use it. A middle approach, which I share, is to substitute another herb in cases of liver disease but to recommend comfrey as part of an herbal therapy for lung diseases, bronchitis, asthma and other respiratory problems.

Echinacea (Echinacea purpurea and E. angustifolia). Echinacea is a bestseller because it works. An antimicrobial herb, which means it has antibiotic properties, echinacea is a popular ingredient in preparations that fight colds and flu. It supports and strengthens the immune system and helps reduce sinus congestion. A specific for colds and flu, especially when taken frequently in large doses at the onset of symptoms, echinacea plays an important supporting role in treating asthma, bronchitis, emphysema, whooping cough, croup, hay fever and other respiratory disorders.

Elder Flowers, Leaves and Berries (Sambucus nigra). The attractive black elder tree has new friends all over the world. Its berries recently made headlines as a cure for the flu, its leaves have expectorant properties and its flowers fight congestion and muscle spasms.

Madeleine Mumcuoglu, an Israeli scientist, developed a syrup made from elderberries that has been shown in clinical tests to prevent and treat influenza. Sambucol syrup and lozenges are sold in health food stores, as is a similar elderberry syrup from the Sambu International Cleansing Program (see appendix for sources). Elder blossoms are a popular ingredient in herbal cough drops such as Ricola lozenges from Switzerland.

Elecampane (Inula belenium). The root or rhizome of this tall medicinal plant is a specific for bronchial coughs, especially in children. This expectorant, antimicrobial plant contains a relaxing mucilage, so that the productive coughing it stimulates is accompanied by a soothing action. Useful in the treatment of asthma and bronchial asthma, elecampane has a history of use in tuberculosis and other respiratory problems.

Elecampane can be blended with other respiratory herbs or used alone. Its bitter principle stimulates digestion and appetite. Do not boil the herb, but brew an infusion by pouring 1 cup boiling water over 1 teaspoon shredded root.

Eyebright (Euphrasia officinalis). This may sound like an herb for the eyes, but it's really a specific for the mucous membranes. An anti-inflammatory astringent herb that fights congestion, eyebright helps clear the sinuses. It can be used alone or added to any herbal preparation for the upper respiratory tract. Brew the tea as an infusion; the recommended tincture dose is 1/2 teaspoon 3 times daily.

Ginger (Zingiber officinale). Ginger is a stimulant, though not so dramatic as cayenne pepper, horseradish, caffeine or Ma huang. Because of its gentle warming influence and its compatibility with all herbs, ginger is an ingredient in many teas blended for respiratory conditions, and its catalyst effect enhances their properties. Ginger is considered safe for people of all ages, from children to the elderly. The dried root should be simmered as a decoction, but fresh ginger root can be shredded or chopped and added to any tea, whether infusion or decoction. Powdered ginger can be used either way as well.

For instructions on making a ginger fomentation (hot compress) to relieve sinus congestion, see page xx.

Goldenrod (Solidago vigaurea). This is Europe's only member of the *Solidago* species, unlike North America, which has several. The European goldenrod, which is far less showy than its American cousins, has a long history of medicinal use. For many herbalists, goldenrod is the herb of choice in treating the chronic inflammation of upper respiratory mucous membranes. It can also be added to other herbs in the treatment of influenza. Brew the tea as an infusion.

Goldenseal (Hydrastis canadensis). A native of North America, goldenseal is one of the world's best-selling medicinal herbs. Most often used to combat bacterial or viral infections or to improve digestion, goldenseal is a specific for sinus congestion and upper respiratory mucus conditions. One of its many plant constituents is berberine, which has been the subject of several scientific investigations. Berberine has antibiotic, antispasmodic and sedative properties, and it stimulates the immune system. Goldenseal is usually added to other herbs, though it can be taken alone. To brew goldenseal tea, make an infusion using 1/2 to 1 teaspoon of the dried root per cup of water and take 3 times daily. A little of the tincture goes a long way; the suggested dose is up to 1/4 teaspoon 3 times daily.

Always buy goldenseal from a reputable source. In the past, goldenseal has been adulterated with turmeric, the bright yellow ingredient in curry powders, and other plants. High-quality goldenseal is expensive because the plant is rare in the wild (it was nearly harvested to extinction in the early 1900s) and difficult to grow.

Not everyone who studies medicinal herbs is enamored of goldenseal; some believe it is overrated, and others warn of its potential toxicity. *Rodale's Illustrated Encyclopedia of Herbs* even concluded, "To be absolutely safe, you should not take goldenseal internally." Large quantities of goldenseal's major component, hydrastine, taken for long periods may produce adverse side effects, but while the theoretical consequences of hydrastine poisoning include respiratory failure, convulsions, miscarriage, the overproduction of white blood cells, depression of the spinal cord and even death, these side effects have not been reported in real life. Considering goldenseal's extraordinary popularity and wide use, most practitioners of herbal medicine consider it safe to use, especially for short periods in the treatment of acute conditions.

Grindelia (*Grindelia spp.*). Grindelia relaxes smooth muscles as well as heart muscles, making it effective in the treatment of bronchitis and asthma when they are linked to rapid heartbeat and nervousness. Grindelia also treats whooping cough and upper respiratory congestion. Because of its relaxing influence on the heart, grindelia may lower blood pressure.

Horehound (*Marrubium vulgare*). Once a popular candy and lozenge ingredient, horehound is a sharply bitter herb with a distinctive flavor. Because of its powerful expectorant properties, horehound is an effective treatment for bronchitis, especially "dry" bronchitis with an unproductive cough. Horehound is an antispasmodic as well as an expectorant, so it soothes and relaxes bronchial muscles while promoting mucus production and its removal.

The plant is so bitter than it's rarely used alone. Dried horehound or its tincture can be added to any herbal tea or syrup. Horehound is probably best known for the cough drops it used to flavor, and while authentic, old-fashioned horehound candy may be hard to find today, it's easy to make your own.

To make horehound candy cough drops, pour 5 cups boiling water over 4 cups loosely packed horehound, or a blend of 2 cups horehound and 2 cups coltsfoot, or a blend of horehound, sage and thyme—or, for that matter, any throat-soothing herbs. Let the tea steep until cool. The tea will be dark, strong and very bitter. Combine 4 cups tea with 4 cups sugar, 1-1/4 cup dark corn syrup and 1 tablespoon butter. Cook these ingredients over high heat until they reach the hard-crack stage (300 to 310 degrees F. on a candy thermometer), which takes quite a while. To test it, place a spoonful of hot syrup in a cup of cold water. At hard crack, the syrup separates into hard, brittle threads as soon as it touches the water. Immediately remove from heat and pour the syrup into two buttered loaf pans or one large pan and, as it cools, score the top for cutting. My scoring isn't always successful, so I sometimes remove the cooled slab of candy from the pan, put it in a heavy plastic bag and whack it with a jam jar to break the pieces apart.

Iceland Moss (Cetraria islandica).

A lichen, Iceland moss has a high mucilage content, making it a soothing demulcent herb in addition to having anti-inflammatory and expectorant properties. These qualities make Iceland moss a specific for bronchitis, sinus congestion and the coughs that accompany colds. Iceland moss requires boiling to make a decoction. Use 1 teaspoon shredded moss per cup of water and simmer, covered, for 20 minutes, or take 1/2 teaspoon tincture 3 times daily.

Irish Moss (Chondrus crispus).

Irish moss isn't a moss at all but rather a seaweed. Its expectorant, demulcent, anti-inflammatory properties made it a traditional therapy for all respiratory conditions, especially bronchitis, irritating coughs, emphysema and other lung conditions. It has a soothing effect on the digestive and urinary systems, and its primary use has always been in the recovery phase of illnesses, when the patient is recuperating from pneumonia, tuberculosis or influenza. The nutritional benefits of Irish moss are important to everyone recovering from serious illness, whether chronic or acute.

To brew a decoction from dried Irish moss, soak 1 tablespoon in 3 cups cold water for 15 minutes or longer. Bring to a boil and simmer, covered, for 20 minutes. To combine Irish moss with other herbs that require boiling (most roots and barks), soak the Irish moss first, then simmer everything together. To add it to herbs that require infusing (most leaves and blossoms), simmer the soaked Irish moss for 20 minutes and remove from heat; take the lid off the pot, add the infusing herbs, replace the cover and let stand 10 to 15 minutes. Strain and serve.

Some Irish moss recipes call for milk instead of water and the addition of sweet spices, such as cinnamon and ginger.

Licorice Root (Glycyrrhiza glabra). Most familiar as an ingredient in black candy ropes and other confections, licorice root is so sweet and aromatic that it's often used to flavor herbal teas. Because of its relaxing effect on the digestive tract, especially the stomach, it is an effective treatment for ulcers. Its expectorant, demulcent, anti-inflammatory and antispasmodic properties make it useful in the treatment of bronchitis, coughs, chest congestion and sore throats. Although it should be simmered as a decoction for best results, shredded licorice root is often an ingredient in teas that are simply infused in hot water. Although licorice tea and tincture can be taken alone, they are often combined with other respiratory herbs. Licorice works well with all of the herbs described here.

Unfortunately, this versatile root has side effects. Glycyrrhizin, its most active principle, can cause edema (fluid retention), heartburn, and, in some people, headaches. These side effects are well documented in German medical texts, for licorice has long been prescribed by that country's physicians for ulcers and stomach pain. One common side effect of licorice overconsumption is a round moon face caused by fluid retention. In Europe, licorice roots are now treated to remove their glycyrrhizin content, but in the U.S. and Canada, the roots are sold untreated. You can, however, purchase deglycyrrhinized licorice capsules, tinctures, and other preparations in health food stores. Because of its effectiveness, deglycyrrhinized licorice is beginning to appear in over-the-counter products for the treatment of heartburn and acid indigestion.

To use licorice for therapeutic purposes, such as the treat-

ment of chronic bronchitis, it is better to take deglycyrrhiz-
ined licorice than to drink large quantities of strongly brewed
tea. A daily cup of beverage-strength licorice root tea isn't
likely to cause problems, but several cups per day could do
so in sensitive people. In small doses and for occasional use,
adverse side effects are unlikely.

Lobelia (*Lobelia inflata*). In his *School of Natural
Healing* Dr. John Christopher wrote, "Lobelia is an efficient
relaxant and is believed to be the best counterirritant known
to mankind. Its action is felt immediately on the serous, mucous, muscular and nervous systems, especially the sympathetic nervous system." The herb causes immediate
relaxation and expansion of the contracted parts of the respiratory system, such as the bronchial tubes, esophagus, glottis
and larynx, making it a specific for nearly every respiratory
condition, especially asthma, emphysema and chest
congestion.

In the early 18th century, lobelia was one of America's
most widely used herbs, thanks to Samuel Thomson, a self-
educated healer who founded his own school of medicine.
Thomsonians, as his followers were called, used lobelia for
every type of illness. Its effects were dramatic, for in the
large doses they recommended, lobelia causes nausea and
vomiting. In fact, one of its common names is pukeweed.

In *Green Pharmacy*, a fascinating history of the evolution
of Western herbal medicine, Barbara Griggs described Thomson's therapy in detail. After vomiting, most patients felt
better and their condition improved. Fevers, colics, quinsies,
dysenteries and chest ailments were medicine's primary complaints then, and the Thomson treatment was outstandingly
successful, especially in contrast to the bleeding and other
practices of orthodox medicine. Thomson became so popular
that the medical establishment of the day brought charges
against him and did its best to discredit the man and his
theories. A similar fate awaited Dr. Albert Coffin, another
lobelia user, in England. More than once, Coffin and lobelia

were put on trial. Much of the testimony condemning lobelia in the 1800s was fabrication, lies told to dishonor Thomson, Coffin and anyone else who recommended it. Lobelia's tarnished reputation survives today, with herbal reference books and FDA reports claiming that it's poisonous, toxic, dangerous and potentially fatal. These accusations, all of which stem from 19th century trials, remain unproven. As Dr. Christopher wrote 150 years after Thomson made lobelia a household word, "The belief that lobelia is a dangerous poison has no basis in fact. . . . Throughout all the prosecutions, there has never been a single instance of harm resulting from the use of lobelia."

According to Mark Blumenthal, executive director of the American Botanical Council and publisher of the journal *HerbalGram* some scientists want to ban lobelia because it causes vomiting, even though, as he notes, "it has nowhere near the toxic potential of aspirin or ibuprofen." Some claim that lobelia causes respiratory distress, but this claim, too, according to Blumenthal, is an untested speculation.

Jethro Kloss, whose *Back to Eden* has been a bestseller since 1939, devoted thirteen pages to lobelia, which he considered a specific for pulmonary complaints such as bronchitis, croup, whooping cough and asthma, and which he called "the most powerful relaxant known among herbs that have no harmful effects."

If you decide to try lobelia, start with small doses of lobelia tincture (7 to 15 drops) in a cup of herbal tea and gradually increase the dosage to 1/8 teaspoon. If you experience nausea or any adverse reaction, reduce the dosage or discontinue use. Lobelia is an important catalyst herb, making the herbal blends in which it is used more effective than they would be without it.

Lobelia is of special interest to smokers, for it helps reduce the craving for tobacco. In addition, it's common name, Indian tobacco, reflects its history as a smoking herb. In addition to their other uses, most herbs can be smoked just like tobacco in pipes or cigarettes. This is a controversial therapy, for some herbalists don't approve of smoking no matter what the product, but many have experienced the bronchiole-relaxing benefits of inhaling the smoke of dried mullein leaves, and a blend of lobelia, coltsfoot and mullein may be a soothing alternative to tobacco.

Lobelia's long and controversial history makes for fascinating reading, and it's well-told by Barbara Griggs, John Christopher and Jethro Kloss. If you have questions about the herb's safety or therapeutic use, please see their books. In addition, write to the Herb Research Foundation for information on lobelia's uses and safety.

Lungwort *(Pulmonaria officinalis)*. As its name suggests, lungwort is an herb for the lungs. A soothing demulcent, expectorant, astringent and anti-inflammatory herb, lungwort has a long history of use in the treatment of coughs and bronchitis. The leaves are brewed as an infusion.

Ma Huang/Ephedra *(Ephedra sinica)*. Ma huang or ephedra is one of 40 related species of primitive, single-stemmed desert bushes. Mormon tea *(E. nevadensis)*, a popular beverage herb in the American Southwest, is another. Unlike Mormon tea, the Chinese species, Ma huang, contains an adrenalin-like stimulant, the alkaloid ephedrine. Ma huang was widely used in the treatment of asthma until it was replaced in Western medicine by its synthetic counterpart, amphetamine, developed in the 1930s under the brand name Benzedrine.

In holistic circles, Ma huang is enjoying a new peak of popularity because it so effectively relieves the symptoms of hay fever, asthma and respiratory distress. It does so by dilating the bronchial tubes, which results in deeper and faster breathing and increased oxygen intake.

Although Ma huang is a natural substance and has fewer side effects than amphetamine, it does have side effects. Ma huang increases blood pressure and pulse rate along with restlessness and nervousness. This is not an herb to take at bedtime—at least, not by itself or in large quantities.

Note that Ma huang is a controversial herb implicated in some sudden deaths, such as heart attacks in young people. Most of these cases involve herbal "speed" products, stimulants promoted as a natural way to get high. Not all herbs are safe in any quantity, as these cases demonstrate. Always use common sense when you use herbs: study their uses and side effects with care.

In response to concerns about ephedra's safety raised by the FDA, the American Herbal Products Association and National Nutritional Foods Association have endorsed warning labels for over-the-counter products that contain Ma huang, stating that users should seek advice from a health care professional if they are pregnant or nursing, have high blood pressure, heart disease, thyroid disease, diabetes or prostate enlargement or take prescription drugs such as MAO inhibitors. The label recommends reducing or discontinuing use if nervousness, tremor, sleeplessness, loss of appetite or nausea occur. This herb should be kept out of the reach of children and is not recommended for children under 13.

Ephedrine stimulants are easily abused. Tolerance to ephedra's stimulant effect builds up quickly with continued use so that larger doses are needed to obtain the same effect and its overuse may weaken the adrenal glands. If you are taking Ma huang, cut down on your consumption of coffee, black or green tea and colas because caffeine taken at the same time will increase nervousness, insomnia, blood pressure and pulse rate.

You will find Ma huang in nearly every herbal hay fever preparation because of its decongestant, antihistamine properties. Capsules, tablets, teas and tinctures combine Ma huang with other herbs, and Ma huang is sold separately as a tea or tincture. One-half to one dropperful of Ma huang tincture produces a strong stimulant effect in most people, lasting for two to four hours.

Marshmallow *(Althaea officinalis)*. The root and leaf of this demulcent, soothing, anti-inflammatory, emollient

and expectorant herb, which is rich in mucilage, make marshmallow a specific for any condition that creates an irritating
cough. The root is most widely used and is often blended
with other herbs in teas, syrups and other preparations for
treating coughs, bronchitis and respiratory congestion.

To make a marshmallow root cough syrup, simmer 1 tablespoon chopped, dried marshmallow root and 1/4 teaspoon cinnamon in 2 cups water for 25 minutes. Strain and recombine
with 2 cups sugar or honey and simmer for 5 to 10 minutes,
stirring well to be sure all the sugar is dissolved. Add 1/4
cup orange juice and pour the syrup into a glass jar that can
be sealed.

Mullein (Verbascum thapsus). Mullein is practically
synonymous with the respiratory system. Introduced to North
America by European settlers, mullein was soon embraced
by native tribes. The Menominees smoked the dried, powdered root for respiratory complaints, other tribes such as the
Mohegans and Penobscots smoked the dried leaves for the
same purpose and the Catawba Indians made a sweetened
syrup from boiled mullein roots for their children's coughs.
When mullein's popularity peaked in 1913, its dried yellow
flowers brought a wholesale price of 80 cents per pound, a
substantial sum. A demulcent herb with anti-inflammatory
properties, mullein is also an expectorant, antispasmodic,
soothing nervine and astringent. Its dried leaves and flowers
tone the respiratory system's mucous membranes, reducing
inflammation and alleviating congestion. Some asthmatics report relief from drinking mullein tea every day, and its dried
leaf can be burned and the smoke inhaled to interrupt asthma
attacks. To brew medicinal strength mullein tea, use 2 teaspoons herb per cup of boiling water, cover and let stand for
10 to 15 minutes, then strain and serve. Or brew a quart of
mullein tea by filling a glass jar with boiling water and 3
tablespoons dried mullein, cover and let stand for 15 minutes,
then pour tea as needed. Heat if desired or serve at room
temperature. Mullein blends well with all of the herbs de-

scribed here and is often one of several herbs used in effective tea or tincture blends.

Mustard (*Brassica alba* or *B. nigra*). The familiar yellow spice does more than flavor hot dogs. As well as clearing the sinuses, it has stimulating external applications. Mustard poultices or plasters are a traditional treatment for chest cold congestion. To make one, spread a paste of powdered mustard seed and water on a cloth and cover the mustard with gauze, then apply the gauze side of this mustard sandwich to the area that needs warming. Remove after a minute and check to see if the skin is reddened. If not, repeat; if so, remove the plaster and apply a thin coat of olive oil.

Few baths are as soothing to cold, aching bones and stuffy sinuses as mustard baths. For a hydrotherapy treat, combine Epsom salts, sea salt, borax (the laundry product) and/or baking soda in any proportions to make a basic bath salt.

In a gallon size Zip-Lock plastic bag, combine 4 cups of the salt mixture with 1 cup powdered mustard. Knead the closed bag to distribute the mustard evenly and break up any lumps in the salt. Add several drops of eucalyptus essential oil or tea tree oil, or add 4 tablespoons of powdered ginger, and mix well. Empty the bag under hot running water and fill the tub to a comfortably warm temperature. Soak for at least 15 to 20 minutes. For best results, pat yourself dry, wrap yourself in blankets (perspiration is desired) and stay warm for half an hour.

Nettle (*Urtica dioica*). An irritating weed that leaves tiny itching blisters wherever it touches, stinging nettle can be the bane of gardeners. But don't let its annoying habits fool you. Nettle can be a hay fever sufferer's best friend. Freeze-dried nettle in capsules taken daily helps prevent allergy symptoms, and the same claim is made for nettle tea and tincture, although they haven't been tested in double-blind clinical trials the way freeze-dried nettle has. In Europe, nettles are a popular spring tonic. Throughout the world, they are respected as a plant that strengthens and supports the entire body. Brew as an infusion for tea. When heated, nettles lose their sting.

Oatgrass *(Avena sativa).* The grass of the common oat is a nutritive tonic for the nervous system and is recommended for nervous exhaustion, irritability, stress and general debility. It can play an important role in the treatment of all respiratory illnesses because it helps the mind and body relax. In addition, oatgrass can help smokers. In 1971, a report by C. Anand, published in the science journal, *Nature,* showed that a tincture of oatgrass significantly reduced the craving for cigarettes in those studied. Oatgrass tincture can be added to any tea or liquid, or it can be placed directly on the tongue. For smokers, the recommended dosage is half a dropperful whenever you crave a cigarette; for other conditions, take 1/2 to 1 teaspoon 3 to 4 times daily.

Osha *(Ligusticum spp.).* Although osha is also called lovage, it should not be confused with the garden plant that resembles celery. Native to the American Southwest, Osha's sharply pungent dried root has a long history of use in the treatment of bronchial coughs. The root can be chewed, brewed as a decoction or used as a tincture. In his *Medicinal Plants of the Pacific West,* Michael Moore recommended osha root "for dry, irritative cough; acute chest cold with dry membranes and fever; and obstinate respiratory virus that doesn't peak properly."

Plantain *(Plantago major).* A familiar lawn and garden weed, plantain is a close cousin of the popular bulking agent, psyllium. A cooling, emollient, mildly astringent, antiseptic and decongestant herb, plantain can be valuable in the treatment of bronchitis and other respiratory complaints. Plantain syrups, made with sugar or honey, are popular European cough treatments.

Pleurisy Root *(Asclepias tuberosa).* As its name implies, pleurisy root is a specific for the lungs and all chest complaints. A bright orange flowering plant popularly known as butterfly weed, pleurisy root aids the removal of congestion while reducing inflammation. It helps to dry and disinfect respiratory passages. A stimulant, expectorant, tonic, antispasmodic and relaxing nervine, pleurisy root has a long history of use in treating pulmonary complaints. Native American tribes boiled the roots for tea or chewed them for this purpose. Prepare the dried root as a decoction or the powdered root as an infusion, using 1 to 2 teaspoons herb per cup of water.

Red Clover (*Trifolium pratense*). The blossoms of this cheerful plant, popular with bees for its sweet nectar, are useful in almost any herbal blend because of their versatile tonic effect. Best known as an alterative or blood purifier, red clover is also an expectorant and antispasmodic, so it helps clear congestion and soothe irritation. Add to any combination of herbs or brew alone, using 1 to 2 teaspoons of herb per cup of boiling water to make an infusion. Use both the tea and tincture generously for bronchitis, irritated coughs, emphysema or asthma.

Sage (*Salvia officinalis*). Sage has so many beneficial uses that for centuries, herbalists have recommended it above most other plants. Its powerful antimicrobial, astringent, antispasmodic, anti-inflammatory properties make sage a specific for inflammation of the upper respiratory tract, and its tea makes an effective gargle for sore throats, laryngitis, pharyngitis and tonsillitis. To prepare sage tea, use 1 to 2 teaspoons of dried leaf per cup of boiling water, cover and let stand 10 minutes. Use hot or warm tea for gargling as often and as long as possible. Sage produces a soothing steam for inhalation.

Slippery Elm Bark (*Ulmus fulva*). Slippery elm bark is the active ingredient in slippery elm lozenges and many cough preparations. A soothing demulcent, emollient herb, slippery elm protects and soothes irritated, inflamed mucous membranes.

Prepare a decoction by mixing 1 part of the powdered herb with 8 to 10 parts water, creating a paste first to prevent lumping. Cover, bring to a boil, simmer over low heat for 15 to 20 minutes, strain and serve. To combine with other roots and barks, prepare as a decoction. To combine with most blossoms or leaves, increase the amount of water to accommodate all of the herbs in use, then prepare the decoction as described above. Remove the pan from heat, add the herbs to be infused, cover and let stand an additional 10 to 15 minutes. Strain and serve.

Sweet Violet *(Viola odorata).* This cheerful plant has been used for centuries as a remedy for coughs and congestion. Its an expectorant, blood cleansing, anti-inflammatory and diuretic herb that can be used alone or added to any combination of herbs for upper respiratory congestion, coughs or bronchitis. Infuse the dried leaves or blossoms.

Thuja *(Thuja occidentalis).* The evergreen also known as Northern White Cedar, thuja is an expectorant, antimicrobial, diuretic, astringent and tonic herb. Its young twigs are used to brew infusion teas for bronchial congestion, though it is not recommended for dry, irritable coughs. Because the essential oil of thuja can be toxic, this herb is not recommended during pregnancy, nor is the distilled essential oil recommended for any internal use. Many North American evergreens have medicinal properties, and the essential oils of thuja, pine, spruce and fir make wonderful room fragrances and facial steam treatments. Spruce gum, the resin of the red spruce, was used by native tribes as a chewing gum and expectorant. Thuja tincture should be used sparingly, up to 1 dropperful 3 times daily, added to tea or other fluids in the treatment of bronchial congestion.

Thyme *(Thymus vulgaris).* This familiar culinary herb has dramatic healing properties similar to those of sage. It can be used as a tea for upper respiratory congestion or as a disinfecting mouthwash or gargle. Thyme tea is often recommended for whooping cough, bronchitis and asthma. Brew as an infusion.

Tea Tree Oil (*Melaleuca alternifolia*). Tea tree oil has become a household word in recent years, thanks to the promotional efforts of Australian tea tree oil producers. The essential oil of Melaleuca applied under the nose or to the chest helps relieve congestion; lozenges and mouthwashes containing the oil soothe sore throats; the oil is a powerful disinfectant and can be used to prevent the growth of mold or bacteria in the reservoirs of humidifiers and dehumidifiers; and a 0.8 percent solution has been shown to kill dust mites.

Wild Cherry Bark (*Prunus serotina*). A familiar cough drop ingredient, wild cherry bark helps prevent congestion, increases expectoration, is an antispasmodic, an antiseptic and a relaxing nervine. Because it sedates the cough reflex, wild cherry bark is useful in treating bronchitis, whooping cough and smoker's cough. The herb can be used in infusions or decoctions.

To make an effective cough syrup, simmer 1 teaspoon wild cherry bark with 2 teaspoons chopped marshmallow root in 2 cups water for 20 minutes. Add 2 cups sugar or honey, stir well and simmer 5 minutes. Pour into a glass jar and seal.

APPENDIX: RESOURCES AND RECOMMENDED READING

The resources listed here are only a few of the hundreds available in the U.S. Because the world of herbal medicine is growing fast, there will be even more by the time you read this.

Herbals and Related References

Christopher, John. *School of Natural Healing*. Springville, Ut.: Christopher Publications, 1978.

Foster, Steven, and James A. Duke. *Peterson Field Guides*: *Eastern/Central Medicinal Plants*. Boston: Houghton Mifflin, 1990. Superior field guide with well-documented medicinal uses.

Grieves, Mrs. M. *A Modern Herbal*. New York: Dover Books, 1971, reprint of 1931 original. A two-volume classic.

Griggs, Barbara. *Green Pharmacy: The History and Evolution of Western Herbal Medicine.* Rochester, Vt.: Healing Arts Press, 1991.

Hoffmann, David. *The Holistic Herbal.* Dorset, England: Element Books, 1983. Popular modern reference.

Keville, Kathi. *The Illustrated Herbal Encyclopedia.* New York: Bantam Doubleday, 1992. Recommended.

Kloss, Jethro. *Back to Eden.* Loma Linda, Calif.: Back to Eden Books, 1988. Updated classic, owned by everyone.

Lust, John. *The Herb Book.* New York: Bantam Books, 1974. Excellent, inexpensive basic herbal.

Mabey, Richard. *The New Age Herbalist.* New York: Collier Books, 1985.

Moore, Michael. *Medicinal Plants of the Pacific West.* Santa Fe: Red Crane Books, 1993.

Murray, Michael, and Joseph Pizzorno. *Encyclopedia of Natural Medicine.* Rocklin, Calif.: Prima Publishing, 1991.

Reader's Digest. *The Magic and Medicine of Plants.* Pleasantville, N.Y.: Reader's Digest Association, 1986. Good overview, some overly cautious warnings.

Rodale's Illustrated Encyclopedia of Herbs. Emmaus, Pa.: Rodale Press, 1987.

Theiss, Barbara and Peter. *The Family Herbal.* Rochester, Vt.: Healing Arts Press, 1989. Introduction to European herbalism, recommended.

Tierra, Michael. *The Way of Herbs.* New York: Pocket Books, 1983. Recommended basic herbal.

Treben, Maria. *Health through God's Pharmacy.* Steyr, Austria: Wilhelm Ennsthaler, 1980.

Weiss, Rodolf Fritz. *Herbal Medicine.* English translation of the sixth German edition, 1988. Imported by Medicina Biologica, Portland, Ore. Excellent reference.

Herbal Magazines

The Herb Companion, 201 East 4th Street, Loveland, Colo. 80537.

The Herb Quarterly, PO Box 689, San Anselmo, Calif. 94960.

HerbalGram, P.O. Box 201660, Austin, Tx. 78720.

Herbal Organizations

American Botanical Council, P.O. Box 201660, Austin, Tx. 78720.

American Herb Association, P.O. Box 1673, Nevada City, Calif. 95959.

American Herbalists Guild, P.O. Box 1683, Sequel, Calif. 95073.

Herb Research Foundation, 1007 Pearl Street, Suite 200, Boulder, Colo. 80302.

Northeast Herbal Association, P.O. Box 479, Milton, N.Y. 12547.

Herbal Education

Directory of Herbal Education, Intra-American Specialties, 3014 N. 400 W., West Lafayette, Ind. 47906. Review of on-site and correspondence courses.

Blazing Star Herbal School by Gail Ulrich, P.O. Box 6, Shelburne Falls, Ma. 01370.

East West Master Course in Herbology by Michael Tierra, P.O. Box 712, Santa Cruz, Calif. 95061.

The Science and Art of Herbalism: A Home Study Course by Rosemary Gladstar, P.O. Box 420, East Barre, Vt. 05649.

Dried Herbs and Teas by Mail

Avena Botanicals, P.O. Box 365, West Rockport, Me. 04865.

Blessed Herbs, 109 Barre Plains Road, Oakham, Me. 01068.

Frontier Cooperative Herbs, P.O. Box 299, Norway, Ia. 52318.

Green Terrestrial, P.O. Box 41, Route 9W, Milton, N.Y. 12547.

The Herb Closet, 104 Main Street, Montpelier, Vt. 05602.

The Herbfarm, 32804 Issaquah Fall City Road, Fall City, Wash. 98024.

Island Herbs, Ryan Drum, Waldron Island, Wash. 98297.

Jean's Greens, 54 McManus Road, Rensselaerville, N.Y. 12147.

Mountain Rose Herbs, Box 2000, Redway, Calif. 95560.

Pacific Botanicals, Catalog Request, 4350 Fish Hatchery Road, Grants Pass, Ore. 97527.

Penzeys, Ltd., merchants of quality spices, P.O. Box 1448, Waukesha, Wi. 43187.

Richters, Goodwood, Ontario L0C 1A0, Canada. Excellent catalog.

Sage Mountain Herb Products, P.O. Box 420, East Barre, Vt. 05649.

Trinity Herbs, P.O. Box 199, Bodega, Calif. 94992.

Wild Weeds, P.O. Box 88, Redway, Calif. 95560.

Hypo-Allergenic Products by Mail

Allergy Control Products, Inc., 96 Danbury Road, Ridgefield, Conn. 06877.

Himalayan Publishers, RR1, P.O. Box 405, Honesdale, Pa. 18431. Neti Pot, ceramic nasal rinse device. Similar products in Self-Care and other catalogs.

National Allergy Supply, 4579 Georgia Highway 120, Duluth, Ga. 30136.

Seventh Generation, 49 Hercules Drive, Colchester, Vt. 05446-1672.

Real Goods, 555 Leslie Street, Ukiah, Calif. 95482-5507.

The Natural Choice, 1365 Rufina Circle, Santa Fe, N.M. 897505.

Self-Care, 5850 Shellmound Street, Emeryville, Calif. 94608-1901.

Special Herbal Products

Flora, Inc., P.O. Box 950, Lynden, Wash. 98264. Sambu International Cleansing Program (elderberry syrup); sold in a health food stores.

J.B. Harris, Inc., 4324 Regency Drive, Glenview, Ill. 60025. Sambucol (elderberry) syrup and lozenges; sold in health food stores.

The Heritage Store, P.O. Box 444, Virginia Beach, Va. 23458-0444. Edgar Cayce remedies by mail.

Home Health Products, 949 Seahawk Circle, Virginia Beach, Va. 23452. Edgar Cayce remedies by mail.

INDEX